ALLERGEN

Edited by **Seyyed Shamsadin Athari**

Allergen
http://dx.doi.org/10.5772/65229
Edited by Seyyed Shamsadin Athari

Contributors

Veronique Schulten, Marcia Nalesso Costa Harder, Valter Arthur, Larissa Nalesso Costa Harder, Ivana Djuric-Filipovic, Zorica Zivkovic, Djordje Filipovic, Gordana Kostic, Snezana Zivanovic, Marco Caminati, Thaís Pacheco-Soares, Olga Machado, Debora Mothe de Campos-Mesquita, Planque Mélanie, Nathalie Gillard, Thierry Arnould, Maria C Jimenez-Martínez, Alberto Salazar, Henry Velazquez-Soto, Julio Ayala-Balboa, John Rojas, Julián Quintero, Gelmy Ciro, Seyyed Shamsadin Athari

Published by InTech

Janeza Trdine 9, 51000 Rijeka, Croatia

Publishing Process Manager Martina Usljebrka
Technical Editor SPi Global
Cover InTech Design team

First published October, 2017
Printed in Croatia
Legal deposit, Croatia: National and University Library in Zagreb

Additional hard copies can be obtained from orders@intechopen.com

Allergen, Edited by Seyyed Shamsadin Athari
p. cm.
Print ISBN 978-953-51-3567-8
Online ISBN 978-953-51-3568-5

For EU product safety concerns:
IN TECH d.o.o., Prolaz Marije Krucifikse Kozulić 3, 51000 Rijeka, Croatia,
info@intechopen.com or visit our website at intechopen.com.

Meet the editor

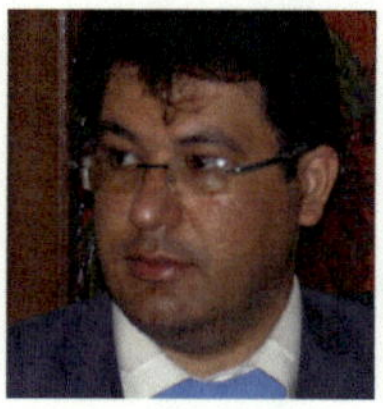

Dr. Seyyed Shamsadin Athari (DVM, MPH, PhD) is an assistant professor of Immunology in the Department of Immunology, Faculty of Medicine, Zanjan University of Medical Sciences, Zanjan, Iran. He has a postdoc in allergy and asthma toxicology and fellowship in asthma management and controlling network. He published more than 60 manuscripts on the international journals in immunology, allergy, and asthma fields and more than 25 books. He is a member of the editorial board of more than 45 international journals in medical sciences.

Contents

Preface

Despite the revolutionary progresses and innovative therapeutic strategies in medical sciences, mankind has encountered some newly emerging diseases and some previously known but apparently more occurring diseases. One of the serious and immune-mediated illnesses is food allergy. There have been frequent reports indicating the alarmingly increase of food allergy incidence particularly in recent decades as a result of extensive ease of access and availability of processed, enriched, or modified foods. Today, a substantial proportion of the industrially produced foods is genetically modified to be more enriched, especially at their protein content. Food proteins are the main cause of the immune sensitization and thereby subsequent development of food allergy.

In light of unraveling the recent advances from an immunologic perspective in the context of the molecular mechanisms involved in establishment of food allergy and providing a comprehensive review yet free of unnecessary complexity and detail, supporting all aspects contributing to the food allergy such as pathophysiology, diagnosis, management, and treatment, I collaborated with a group of the eminent experts in the field of immunology, immunotherapy, analytic, and diagnostic methods and food technology to write a book concisely covering the mentioned topics. I organized the chapters logically from the basics to the deeply mechanistic viewpoint to the advanced diagnostic approaches and finally to the managerial and therapeutic strategies. Efforts have been made on each chapter to precisely provide the compendious yet comprehensive information on its topic. I have frequently faced with probing questions during my research and teaching experiences particularly by students who confused by the paradoxical functions of immune system which leads the immunologic responses towards the sensitization in some people, ignoring the potential food allergens in some other people. I think this book can answer these intricacies and help the students for understanding the exact immunological pathways involved in food allergy. Moreover, the material covered in the book stands on its own manner of simplicity but comprehensiveness making it distinct from other books in this field of science. In addition, this book benefits from a superiority of providing the most recent advances to better understand the molecular pathways contributing to the food allergy. I have also written a brief intro simply describing the food allergy basics, definitions, its difference with food intolerance, and most effective treatment methods.

This book is written in an easy and readable way, appropriate for both undergraduate and postgraduate students of biology and medicine. However, the book is also intended to provide an advanced knowledge and recent progresses in the field of food allergy appropriate for academic researchers, immunologists, physicians, and clinical specialists. Because of its simplicity and briefness, it can be used also as a guidebook in hospitals or laboratories, providing the most usual diagnostic and treatment methods.

I would like to extend special thanks to Ms Martina Ušljebrka for her kind assistance for organizing and skillfully editing the text of the book. I would also like to acknowledge Professor Mostafa Moin for his valuable comments and guidance in the completion of this book.

Dr. Seyyed Shamsadin Athari
Department of Immunology,
Faculty of Medicine,
Zanjan University of Medical Sciences,
Zanjan, Iran

Chapter 1

Introductory Chapter

Seyyed Shamsadin Athari and Ghasem Vahedi

Additional information is available at the end of the chapter

http://dx.doi.org/10.5772/intechopen.70176

1. Introduction

Recently, a clear definition was provided by National Institute of Allergy and Infectious Diseases (NIAID) for the food allergy in which it is defined as the usually an extreme immune response against the specific proteins in food. The immune reactions triggered by these allergenic proteins are started immediately after consuming an allergic food or lately after 2–3 days. The immune response can be acute and deadly in some cases and happens in minutes, causing angioedema, throat or tongue swelling, obstruction of respiratory airways secondary to swelling, and rapid fall of blood pressure, which are indicative of a dangerous life-threatening immune reaction called anaphylaxis. The only way to effectively control an anaphylaxis shock is to give an epinephrine (adrenaline) shot to the patient as soon as possible. But some common symptoms which the patients with food allergy experience after an allergen challenge are moderate, including gastrointestinal hypersensitivity, urticaria, itchy rashes, edema in different tissues/organs, rhinitis, and chronic asthma-like reactions.

However, one should bear in mind that the food allergy is differed by its mechanism of action and the initial factors involved in the onset of the symptoms from the food intolerance. The food allergy is generally an IgE-mediated immune response but food intolerance is a difficulty in digesting a specific food or compound within a food. For instance, some people cannot digest lactose, which is usually found in milk, because they have insufficient or no activity of lactase or suffer from completely absence of the lactase, an enzyme that breaks lactose to smaller carbohydrates. This is a typical food intolerance, which is unrelated to the immune system and in comparison to reactions triggered by food allergy, and is characterized by less acute clinical manifestations such as stomach ache, headache, irritable bowel, hives (urticaria), cough, runny nose, and feeling unwell.

Food allergy is more frequent among children than in adults by which most cases of food allergy occur during first 5 years of life and disappear later spontaneously. It was proposed that the patients, who the onset of symptoms occurs in earlier ages, are more likely to maintain their allergy to foods until their later ages. The cow's milk, peanuts, and tree nuts are three most usual causes of food allergy among children while shellfish, fruits, and vegetables are three most common causes of the food allergy among adults. However, millions of people involved in food allergy worldwide in which the globalization, transportation of new foods to the nonnative countries, increased consuming of processed foods, and production of enriched foods by food-derived proteins such as gluten or the soy proteins are the factors supporting the increasing trend of food allergy. Based on epidemiologic studies, the overall prevalence of food allergy varies between 1 and 10% of the population. In a survey based on tens of thousands medical records in the USA, the prevalence of food allergy estimated 8% among children, 3% of which experience severe immune responses. In the USA, about 12 millions of people have a type of food allergy. Surprisingly, despite the substantial progress in our knowledge about healthy nutrition and, therefore, noticeable improvements in the health and hygiene standards of the food processing and enrichments, the prevalence of food allergy has been increased continuously in recent years. In the USA, the prevalence of food allergy among children aged 0–17 has been increased from 3.4% in 1997–1999 to 5.1% in 2009–2011, showing a 50% increase in frequency. In this regard, the food allergy is not a simple and negligible health issue by considering the fact that it can impose the heavy costs to the national health budget. In the USA, the healthcare system pays annual $24.8 billion for the food allergy.

The pathogenesis of allergic responses in food-sensitive patients from an immunologic perspective is relatively well characterized in recent years but the precise primary mechanism which initiates the immune reaction against some allergenic proteins within foods in some people but not in others remains to be elucidated. Food allergies can be classified into three main categories based on their primary mechanism of initiation including 1. The pathogenic and allergic responses by which mediated by IgE production, 2. The responses which is composed of the mixed IgE- and T cells-mediated reactions, and 3. The allergic reactions unrelated to the IgE production and mediated by allergen-specific T cells.

Generally, food allergy can be considered as the atopic disorder. Progression of atopic disorders is occurred first during infancy or early childhood, clinically is being manifested as the atopic dermatitis, in a form of a phenomenon called atopic march. The emergence of an atopic disease (such as atopic dermatitis) in a patient has been associated tightly with the later progression of allergic disorders such as food allergy, allergic rhinitis, and allergic asthma. Furthermore, nonatopic illnesses such as celiac/coeliac disease or gluten sensitivity are being initiated by the completely distinct mechanisms, although again the immune system is involved. In fact, celiac disease or gluten sensitivity is a type of food intolerance not food allergy in which IgE has no role in their pathogenesis but other antibodies such as IgA and IgG does. In celiac disease, delayed cell-mediated hypersensitivity drives the immune system reactions in small intestine after digesting a gluten-containing food by a genetically predisposed individual, causing the chronic intestinal inflammation and enteropathy that result in leaky gut. However, the abnormal mixed IgE- and cell-mediated immune responses are responsible for 14–37% cases of the food allergy, making this category the most frequent type of the food allergy. The food allergies with the IgE as the only causative mechanism comprise 0.4–10% of the food-allergic cases, ranked as the second prevalent type of food allergy.

IgE-mediated immune responses usually occur rapidly in minutes and causes severe and acute clinical manifestations. However, this type of food allergy varies in different countries in order to the type of the food responsible for allergenic reactions. In most of the Asian countries, shellfish is the most frequent cause of the food allergy, whereas the wheat allergy is infrequent. Initially, food-sensitized individuals, in their subsequent exposure to that food, experience severe and immediate responses that are driven by IgE. Food allergen-specific IgE molecules are attached to the specific receptors on the effector cells such as basophils and mast cells then the allergens can bind to these receptor-bound IgE molecules, leading the cells for degranulation and release of abundant amounts of inflammatory mediators such as histamine, TNF-α, IL-4, and IL-13. Histamine is one of the key mediators in IgE-mediated allergic responses, makes the capillaries permeable to the immune cells, causes the broncho-constriction, smooth muscle cells contraction, mucus release, and urticaria and has a key role in initiating the anaphylaxis. Mast cells contribute not only in the immediate phase of allergic responses by mass-degranulation of their inflammatory mediators like histamine and serotonin but also contribute in late-phase immune response by cytokine production, antigen presenting, and T cell priming. After an immediate phase of allergic response against an allergen food, the later phase of immune response is triggered and maintained by production of leukotrienes and cytokines such as IL-4, IL-5, and IL-13. A broad range of organ-specific and systemic clinical manifestations occur during an IgE-mediated allergic response against an allergen food. The organ-specific manifestations comprise the gastrointestinal, oral, skin, and respiratory symptoms, while the systemic manifestations include hypotension, hypothermia, and anaphylactic reactions.

Mixed immune pathways-mediated food allergy is frequently occurred in food allergen-sensitized individuals, characterized by atopic symptoms which are mostly the exacerbated atopic dermatitis after exposure to an allergenic food or in some cases gastrointestinal allergic reactions such as eosinophilic oesophagitis. The immune system in mixed food allergies acts through both IgE-mediated pathway and cell-mediated delayed hypersensitivity. The activation of T helper 2 (T_H2) cells has a central role in triggering the delayed hypersensitivity against allergenic foods.

The last type of the food allergy is mediated through non-IgE-related pathways, largely driven by the action of allergen-specific T cells. In non-IgE-mediated food allergy, (initiated by allergen-specific T cells), the most common clinical symptoms are more occurred within the gastrointestinal tract rather than in other organs such as respiratory system or skin. Generally, infants and toddlers are involved in this type of food allergy, which results in some specific types of enteropathy and enteric inflammation such as the food protein-induced enterocolitis syndrome, food protein-induced proctocolitis, and food protein enteropathy, and their etiologies have been remained unknown to date.

As an alternative viewpoint, regarding the time required for onset of symptoms, the food allergies can be classified into two groups including those mediated by rapid immune responses in which the mast cells, basophils, and IgE play main role and those mediated by delayed immune responses in which the basophils, T cells, and eosinophils are responsible for chronic allergic inflammation and late-phase immune reactions.

However, the mechanism by which the host's immune system develops the tolerance (healthy reaction) or sensitization (allergy) against a food has been partially elucidated. A subtype of dendritic cells (DCs) classified as the $CD103^+$ DCs are the key cells concerting the immune system tune against the food allergens, leading the immune responses either toward a tuned (healthy) or a false response (allergy). DCs sample the food allergens thorough the epithelial cell barrier of the gut. Other antigen presenting cells such as macrophages help the DCs for antigen sampling. Then these antigen activated DCs migrate from the lamina propria toward a secondary lymphoid tissue and there prime the naïve T lymphocytes to differentiate into $FOXP3^+$ regulatory T (T_{reg}) cells. These primed and antigen-specific T_{reg} cells are main immune cells responsible for tolerance against food allergens. In addition, $CD103^+$ DCs also involved in triggering the naïve $CD4^+$ T cell to polarize into $FOXP3^-$, IL-10-secreting T cells which are called type 1 regulatory T cells (Tr1 cells). Tr1 cells have also critical role in dampening the immune response against food antigens. The DC-mediated polarized T cells contribute in suppressing the immune reaction against food allergens and induce the IgA production by B cells. In contrast, during the sensitization process, $CD103^+$ DCs shift the immune system toward a cascade of responses directed by T_H2 cells. In sensitized patients, the food allergens trigger inflammatory responses mediated by gut epithelial cells via producing the thymic stromal lymphopoietin (TSLP), IL-25, and IL-33. These cytokines affect the DCs, empowering them to deviate the polarization of naïve T cells toward the T_H2 cells rather than the T_H1 cells. Then T_H2 cells induce the class-switching of B cells to produce allergen-specific IgE followed by subsequent responses by effector cells (mast cells, basophils) which is end in the food allergy.

There have been a series of diagnostic methods, some of them developed decades ago but until recently have been remained reliable enough although in some cases they give false positive or false negative result. However, the medical history and physical examination are the first line approach for medical diagnosis of food allergy in which some disorders such as the history of an atopic disease can guide the physician toward a proper diagnosis. In addition, a method based on step-by-step removing the nonallergic food from the dietary regimen until reaching the food causing the allergic response is the only fully reliable method of identifying the original cause of the food allergy. An accurate and generally accepted variant of the method called oral food challenge (OFC) has been developed but it could not be used extensively thus far due to requirement of intensive laboratory resources, its time-consuming procedures and the risk of undergoing anaphylactic reactions. The serologic tests such as measuring the total IgE and allergen-specific IgE, skin tests such as skin prick test, intradermal skin test, and atopy patch test can also help for diagnosis, though these tests indicate only the sensitization not a clinical food allergy. There are also two novel highly accurate diagnostic tests including the component-resolved diagnosis and basophil activation test although yet are being in the developing process in research settings.

The management and treatment methods for food allergy are mostly based on avoidance or elimination of the allergenic food from the dietary regimen. Currently, the only method whose effect can last for long time is known as the allergen-specific immunotherapy (SIT). In the SIT method, the allergen food is usually administered orally to the patient in a controlled manner in order to relieve the food allergy, which is called antigen desensitization. However,

http://dx.doi.org/10.5772/intechopen.70176

other desensitizing immunotherapy methods are also developed and done by introducing the allergen food to the immune system via other routes of administration like sublingual or skin. In the sublingual immunotherapy (SLIT) method, first, a very small amount of the allergen food is placed under the tongue, maintained for minutes then the amount of allergen is increased gradually over the several days or weeks. The results of using SLIT or oral immunotherapy (OIT) have been very promising, making the immune system tolerant to the allergen food in gram amounts. Other therapies mainly relied on mitigating the symptoms such as the anti-IgE monoclonal antibodies, anti-histamines, anti-leukotrienes, and epinephrine. For targeting the non-IgE-mediated but T-cell-dependent food allergies, there are also some symptomatic treatments such as the steroids and anti-IL5, inhibiting the T cells activation. In additidon, some studies suggest that the early introduction of potentially allergenic food may prohibit or decrease the chance for emergence of food allergy. Other studies suggest also a preventive and protective role of vitamin D against food allergy.

Author details

Seyyed Shamsadin Athari[1*], Ghasem Vahedi[2]

*Address all correspondence to: ss.athari@gmail.com and ss.athari@zums.ac.ir

1 Department of Immunology, Faculty of Medicine, Zanjan University of Medical Sciences, Zanjan, Iran

2 Research Center for Food Hygiene and Safety, Shahid Sadoughi University of Medical Sciences, Yazd, Iran

Chapter 2

Food Allergen Analysis: Detection, Quantification and Validation by Mass Spectrometry

Mélanie Planque, Thierry Arnould and
Nathalie Gillard

Additional information is available at the end of the chapter

http://dx.doi.org/10.5772/intechopen.69361

Abstract

Worldwide, food-allergy-related diseases are a significant health problem. While the food industry works on managing cross-contaminations and while clinicians deal with treatment, laboratories must develop efficient analytical methods to ensure detection of hidden allergens that can cause severe adverse reactions. Over the past few years, huge progress has been made in mass spectrometry for the analysis of allergens in incurred and processed foodstuffs, especially as regards sample preparation and enrichment (solid phase extraction, protein precipitation and ultrafiltration). These achievements make it possible to meet the Allergen Bureau's Voluntary Incidental Trace Allergen Labelling (VITAL) sensitivity criteria. The present chapter details the different steps in the development of mass spectrometry methods, from peptide selection to the validation of qualitative and quantitative methods. The chapter focuses mainly on studies performed with incurred and processed food samples to ensure the applicability of the methods to allergen detection in real food products.

Keywords: allergens, advances, detection, quantification, challenges, mass spectrometry, UHPLC-MS/MS, validation

1. Introduction

Food allergies have increased significantly, affecting between 3 and 4% of adults and at least 6% of children [1]. According to the European Academy of Allergology and Clinical Immunology (EAACI), the prevalence of food allergy has doubled over the past 10 years [2]. After an adverse reaction to a foodstuff, which may range from mild to severe (e.g.

anaphylaxis) [3, 4], allergic patients have to exclude that foodstuff from their diet. Each year in the United States, some 100 deaths are caused by anaphylaxis due to food allergy [5], the main culprits being allergens from peanut, tree nuts, fish, shellfish and milk [6]. Currently, there exist no treatments for food allergy, but clinical trials have been performed to test subcutaneous immunotherapy and oral immunotherapy used to desensitize patients [7]. The high level of adverse reactions observed in these trials has led clinicians to find safer alternative therapies, such as sublingual and epicutaneous immunotherapy. These approaches consist, respectively, in placing allergens (drops or tablets) under the tongue or in using a skin patch to induce sustained protection against anaphylaxis [8]. Although they do not treat allergic disease, they improve considerably the quality of life of highly allergic patients and constitute a real hope for them [9, 10]. The number of potentially allergenic ingredients that must appear on food labels differs in different parts of the world [11]. In Europe, regulation (EU) 1169/2011 imposes indicating the following 14 ingredients: milk, peanut, egg, soybean, fish, crustaceans, cereals containing gluten, tree nuts, celery, lupin, mustard, sesame, molluscs and sulfur dioxide [12]. This regulation fails to take into account the accidental introduction of allergens during production, transportation or storage, even though allergens introduced in this manner can trigger severe reactions [13–15]. To protect food consumers, the industry has widely used precautionary allergen labelling (PAL) (i.e. statements such as 'may contain', 'may contain traces of…') [16]. Yet, the lack of correlation between the presence of allergens and precautionary labelling has led customers to lose trust in food labels [17–20]. In a study of food product recalls over a four-year period in the European Union, the United States, Canada, Hong Kong, Australia and New Zealand, 42–90% of the recalls, depending on the country, were justified by the presence of allergens not indicated on the label [21]. Between 2007 and 2012, the Food and Drug Administration (FDA) recalled 732 products because of allergen contaminations [22] and allergic reactions are due to five foods: milk, egg, peanuts, wheat and soybean (**Figure 1**).

The distribution of these recalls in the European Union, reported in **Figure 2**, shows that the products most commonly involved in food recalls are cereals and bakery products.

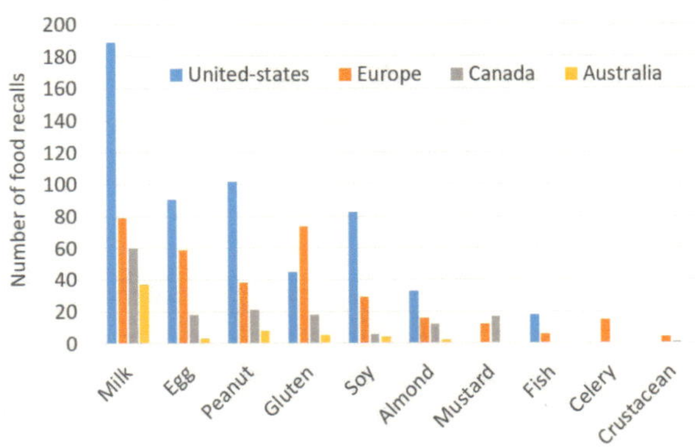

Figure 1. Number of food recalls per allergen category in the United States, Europe, Canada, and Australia between 2012 and 2015 [23–26].

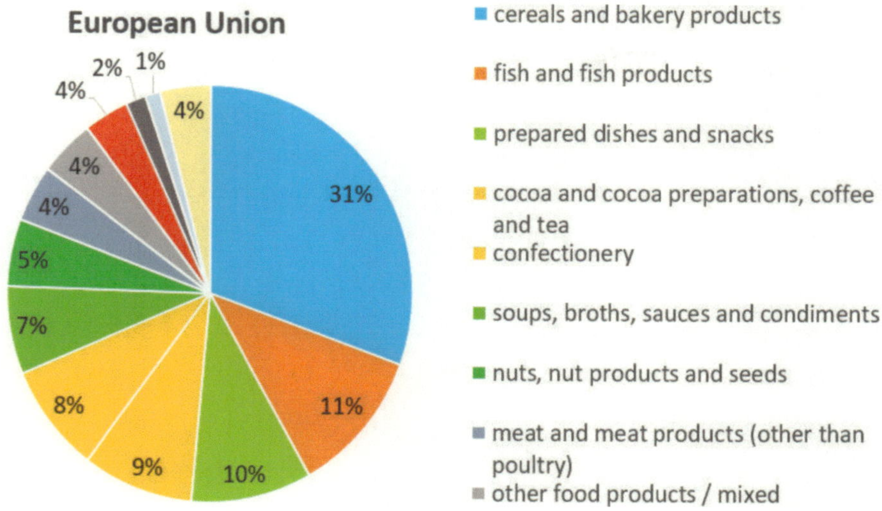

Figure 2. Percentage distribution of food allergen recalls in the European Union (according to the Rapid Alert System for Food and Feed) [24].

The widespread use of PAL can be explained by the lack of regulatory thresholds and the complexity of food allergen management through the supply chain. To counter this lack, the Voluntary Incidental Trace Allergen Labelling (VITAL) system has been developed in Australia and New Zealand to assist food producers in managing cross-contaminations during food production [27]. This system sets allergen thresholds, based on clinical studies, for the protection of 95–99% of the allergic population. Other referentials for allergen thresholds are the European Academy of Allergy and Clinical Immunology (EAACI) and the Netherlands Food and Consumer Product Safety Authority (NVWA) [28] (**Table 1**).

While the systems just mentioned have no regulatory value, food laboratories use them in evaluating method sensitivity. To obtain a concentration expressed in 'mg proteins per kilogram', a food portion size must be considered in order to compare the analytical method with VITAL thresholds (e.g. a portion size of 50 g, **Table 1**). Yet while VITAL thresholds are expressed in 'mg proteins', laboratories express their results in 'mg ingredients' [29, 30] or may refer either to soluble proteins [31, 32] or total proteins [33] per kg. To compare method performances, a conversion factor must thus be applied (e.g. 25% proteins in whole peanuts [34]). Moreover, VITAL action levels have been determined from clinical studies, mostly on the basis of the allergenicity of raw ingredients, although studies have demonstrated a major decrease in allergenicity in baked products. For example, 50–85% of allergic children are able to tolerate baked egg [35] and a study published in 2015 found 63% to tolerate 3.8 g egg-white protein in baked-egg products [36].

Nevertheless, the prevalence of baked product recalls confirms that laboratories must develop sensitive methods for detecting allergens in processed foodstuffs. The most widely used methods are based on the recognition of allergen proteins by antibodies, notably lateral flow device methods and enzyme-linked immunosorbent assays (ELISAs) [39]. DNA-based meth-

Food	Reference dose VITAL (mg of proteins) [27, 34, 37]	Reference dose IEAACI (mg of proteins) [38]	Reference dose NVWA (mg of proteins) [28]	Reference dose VITAL (mg of proteins per kg) Portion size: 50 g
Peanut	0.2	0.2	0.015	4
Cow milk	0.1	0.1	0.016	2
Egg	0.03	0.03	0.0043	0.6
Hazelnut	0.1	0.1	0.011	4
Soy	1.0	1.0	0.078	20
Wheat	1.0	1.0	0.14	20
Cashew	2.0	2.0	1.4	40
Mustard	0.05	0.05	0.022	1
Lupin	4.0	4.0	0.83	80
Sesame	0.2	0.2	0.10	4
Shrimp	10	10.0	3.7	200
Fish	/	0.1	/	/

Table 1. VITAL (http://allergenbureau.net/vital/), EAACI (http://www.eaaci.org/) and NVWA (https://www.nvwa.nl/) reference doses for different food allergens.

ods such as those exploiting the real-time polymerase chain reaction (PCR) [40] are also used to detect the presence of allergens. Currently, mass spectrometry is becoming an alternative to these methods, as heat-processing induces protein denaturation and structural modifications that might result in non-recognition of the target protein by conformational antibodies and thus in the case of ELISAs, lead to false negatives or at least major underestimation of allergen content [41–44]. Mass spectrometry has the advantage of permitting simultaneous analyses for several allergens in food, including processed food products, with high sensitivity and specificity.

This chapter highlights the important improvements made over the last 10 years in mass spectrometry applied to the development of allergen detection methods. It covers and discusses the mass spectrometry methods currently used to detect and quantify allergens in processed food products, including their validation.

2. Detecting food allergens

2.1. Selecting marker peptides

Food allergens (except sulfites) are proteins that need to be digested by enzymes (trypsin and chymotrypsin) so as to generate peptides suitable for routine mass spectrometry analysis. Identification and selection of robust peptides are generally done first on digested raw ingredients before analysis of digested processed ingredients in food matrices. This section summarizes two approaches commonly used to select marker peptides (the instrumental approach and the *in silico* approach) and the specificity and sensitivity critera used.

2.1.1. *Peptide selection*

2.1.1.1. *Instrumental peptide selection*

The first approach is to identify abundant marker peptides by high resolution mass spectrometry (HRMS). Downstream from allergen analysis by HRMS, the generated data are transferred into an algorithm for assigning peptides to MS/MS spectra (MASCOT, X!Tandem, SEQUEST) [45]. For example, Sealey-Voyksner et al. analysed 12 tree nuts and peanut-raw and roasted (176.7°C, 30 min) by time of flight (q-TOF) (Agilent 6530) spectrometry and selected two abundant peptides per tree nut and four for peanut [46]. In a previous study, ice cream spiked with peanuts was analysed by q-TOF (Waters Micromass II) to identify peptides of the Ara h1 allergen [47]. In a 2012 study, Cucu et al. identified several soybean marker peptides by matrix-assisted laser desorption ionization (MALDI-TOF/MS) [48]. The main advantage of this approach is that global peptide and protein profiles can be analysed for the different samples.

2.1.1.2. *In silico peptide selection*

Another strategy for selecting marker peptides is to retrieve target protein sequences from a database, e.g. Uniprot (http://www.uniprot.org/), and to perform an *in silico* digestion with an open access software, e.g. Skyline or MRMaid [49, 50] (**Figure 3**).

In silico digestion with multiple reaction monitoring (MRM) involves generating a list of criteria that must be applied or set by the user as regards peptides, transitions and MS/MS

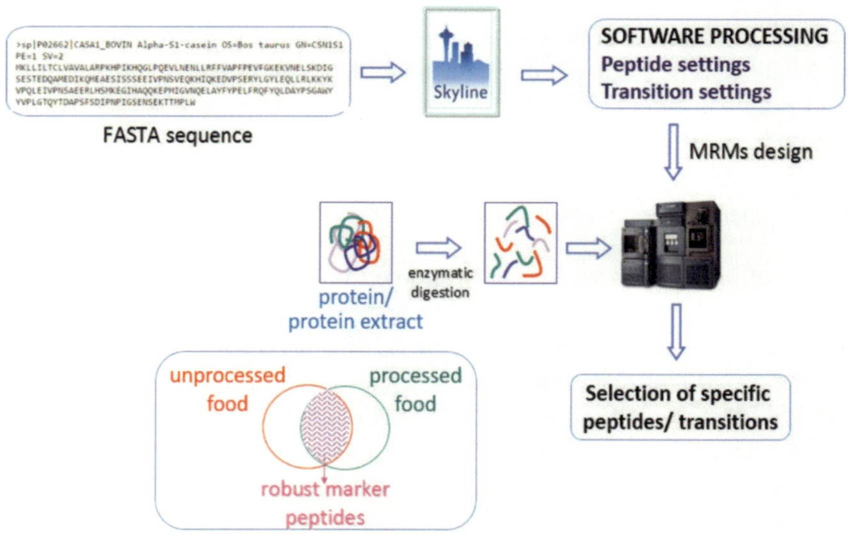

Figure 3. *In silico* peptide selection with the Uniprot database and Skyline software.

parameters (e.g. peptide length, charge states, fragmentation and enzyme). Then raw ingredients or incurred matrices can be analysed by ultra-high performance liquid chromatography coupled to tandem mass spectrometry (UHPLC-MS/MS). This approach allows identification of abundant peptides. It was used by Rogniaux et al. for the analysis of wheat varieties: several gluten peptides were identified with a linear ion trap quadrupole mass filter in tandem with an orbitrap (Thermo Fisher Scientific) [51].

An *in silico* approach also requires a complete database with available protein sequences. Uniprot inventories, however, can be too large (e.g. >145,000 proteins for the wheat species-*Triticum aestivum*), making it necessary to first select target proteins from the literature. Use of a routine UHPLC-MS/MS instrument is the main advantage of the *in silico* approach for laboratories unwilling to invest in a high-resolution mass spectrometer.

2.1.2. Specificity

BLAST: After this selection, blasting must be performed to guarantee the specificity of marker peptides. This step is mandatory but not always included in method development. In one study, for example, Hoofnagle et al. selected five peptides for the detection of β-casein in cookies: EMPFPK (6AA), VLPVPQK (7AA), AVPYPQR (7AA), GPFPIIV (7AA) and DMPIQAFLLYQEPVLGPVR (19AA) [52]. Only one of these peptides could be blasted, and this peptide is 100% homologous to goat, zebu, buffalo, yak and sheep β-casein (Uniprot). In proteomics, peptide blasting should be systematic, even though the international trade frequently introduces new food products and although some proteins can still be missing in the different databases.

The **specificity of selected fragments** is also paramount. To improve specificity, the mass-to-charge ratio (m/z) of the precursor should be lower than the m/z of the fragments. Too-small fragments should be avoided. At least, fragments of 1 to 2 amino acids (b1, b2, y1, y2) should be excluded, which is not always the case in published methods [53, 54].

Blanks: Matrices without allergens must also be analysed to ensure the specificity of the selected transitions of the target peptides. As databases do not cover all possible proteins and as new food products enter the food chain regularly, this experimental testing is crucial to proving method specificity.

2.1.3. Identifying marker peptides in incurred foodstuffs

The advantage of using mass spectrometry is detection of allergens in industrial food products. For such applications, only target peptides and proteins that will be detected in incurred and processed matrices, such as those listed in **Table 2**, need to be retained in the analytical methods. Some peptides are common to the majority of published methods: FFVAPFPEVFGK and YLGYLEQLLR (Casein αS1), and GGLEPINFQTAADQAR (ovalbumin), among others. Target peptides detected after different extraction and purification steps in several types of matrices constitute potential marker peptides for the detection of allergens in a wide variety of foodstuffs.

Authors	Matrix	Allergen	Protein	Peptide	Fragments
Heick et al. [53]	Bread (60 min, 200°C)	Milk	αS1-casein	YLGYLEQLLR	b2, y8
				FFVAPFPEVFGK	y8, y9
			αS2-casein	NAVPITPTLNR	b2, y8
				FALPQYLK	a1, y5
		Egg	Ovalbumin	HIATNAVLFFGR	a2, y10
				YPILPEYLQCVK	y6, y8
				DILNQITKPNDVYSFSLASR	a2, y8
				ELINSWVESQTNGIIR	y9, y10
		Soy	Glycinin	NLQGENEGEDKGAIVTVK	a2, b3
				VFDGELQEGR	a2, y8
				SQSDNFEYVSFK	y3, y10
				EAFGVNMQIVR	y6, y8
		Peanut	Ara h1	DLAFPGSGEQVEK	a3, y9
				GTGNLELVAVR	y5, y6
			Ara h3/4	RPFYSNAPQEIFIQQGR	y6, b7
				WLGLSAEYGNLYR	a2, y11
		Hazelnut	11S globulin	ADIYTEQVGR	y6, y7
				INTVNSNTLPVLR	y4, y9
				QGQVLTIPQNFAVAK	y8, y10
				ALPDDVLANAFQISR	y8, y9
		Walnut	Jug r1	DLPNECGISSQR	y4, y10
				QCCQQLSQMDEQCQCEGLR	y3, y10
				GEEMEEMVQSAR	y7, y8
		Almond	Prunin	GNLDFVQPPR	y3, y7
				GVLGAVFSGCPETFEESQQSSQQGR	y6, y7
				ALPDEVLANAYQISR	y8, y9
				NGLHLPSYSNAPQLIYIVQGR	y6, b11
Pilolli et al. 2016 [56]	Cookie (200°C, 12 min)	Milk	αS1-casein	FFVAPFPEVFGK	y8, y9, y10
				YLGYLEQLLR	y5, y6, y8
		Egg	Ovalbumin	GGLEPINFQTAADQAR	y7, y10, y12
				YPILPEYLQCVK	b4, y8, y9
		Peanut	Conarachin	VLLEENAGGEQEER	y7, y8, y12
				EGEQEWGTPGSEVR	y6, y8, y9

Authors	Matrix	Allergen	Protein	Peptide	Fragments
		Soy	Glycinin G1-G2	SQSDNFEYVSFK	y3, y10
				FYLAGNQEQEFLK	y9, y10, y11
		Hazelnut	11S globulin-like protein	ADIYTEQVGR	y6, y7
				ALPDDVLANAFQISR	y7, y8, y13
Lamberti et al. [57]	Cookie (180°C, 10 min)	Milk	αS1-casein	YLGYLEQLLR	y8, y9, y10
				FFVAPFPEVFGK	y8, y9, y10
				HQGLPQEVLNENLLR	y11, y12
Pedreschi et al. [58]	Cookie (180°C, 16 min)	Peanut	Ara h1	VLLEENAGGEQEER	y9, y8, y7, y6, y4, y2
				DLAFPGSGEQVEK	y10, y9, y8, b4, b3, b2
			Ara h2	CCNELNEFENNQR	y8, y6, y5, y4
				NLPQQCGLR	y7, y6, y5, a2
				CDLEVESGGR	y8, y6, y5, y4
				CMCEALQQIMENQSDR	y14, y11, y10, y8, y7, y6, y5, b2
			Ara h3	LNAQRPDNR	ymax, y8, y7, y5, b2
				SPDIYNPQAGSLK	ymax, y12, y9, y8, y7, y5, b3
				AHVQVVDSNGNR	b7, y6, b5
Huschek et al. [59]	Cookie (190°C, 13 min)	Soy	Gly m6	VFDGELQEGR	903.6/ 489.2/ 788.5
				LSAEFGLR	432.3/ 779.4/ 579.3
				LNALKPDNR	742.4/ 629.3/ 501.2
		Sesame	Ses i6	ISGAQPSLR	472.3/ 728.4/ 671.4
				AFYLAGGVPR	556.3/ 485.3/ 669.4
				SPLAGYTSVIR	795.4/ 866.5/ 575.4
		Lupine	β-conglutin	LLGFGINADENQR	846.4/661.3/ 797.4
				NTLEATFNTR	951.5/838.4/ 709.4
				NPYHFSSQR	761.4/ 624.3/ 477.2

Table 2a. List of target marker peptides used to detect several allergens in bread and cookies [55–59].

2.2. Developing mass spectrometry methods

After selection of marker peptides, the developed method must be able to detect traces of the allergen proteins in the 'mg allergen proteins per kg food product' range. The real chal-

Authors	Matrix	Allergen	Protein	Peptide	Fragments
Planque et al. [33, 60]	Cookie (180°C—18 min), sauce (95°C, 45 min), ice cream and chocolate	Milk	αS1-Casein	FFVAPFPEVFGK	y6, y8, y9
				HQGLPQEVLNENLLR	b4, y6, y7
				YLGYLEQLLR	y5, y6, y7
			αS2-casein	NAVPITPTLNR	b3, y8, y8
			β-lactoglobulin	VYVEELKPTPEGDLEILLQK	y11, y14, y16
				VLVLDTDYK	y5, y6, y7
				LSFNPTQLEEQCHI	y7, y10, y10
		Egg	Ovalbumin	GGLEPINFQTAADQAR	y10, y12, y12
				LTEWTSSNVM EER	y7, y8, y9
				ISQAVHAAHAEINEAGR	y9, y10, y11
			Vitellogenin	EALQPIHDLADEAISR	y6, y7, y12
				NIPFAEYPTYK	y4, y9, y9
				NIGELGVEK	y5, y6, y7
				YLLDLLPAAASHR	y7, y7, y11
			Apovitellenin	NFLINETAR	y5, y6, y7
		Peanut	Cupin	NTLEAAFNAEFNEIR	y7, y8, y9
				RPFYSNAPQEIFIQQGR	b7, y6, y10
				FNLAGNHEQEFLR	y5, y9, y10
				TANELNLLILR	y6, y7, y8
		Soy	Glycinin	ISTLNSLTLPALR	y7, y8, y9
				EAFGVNMQIVR	y5, y6, y7
				ELINLATMCR	y5, y6, y8
				LITLAIPVNKPGR	y7, y9, y11
Parker et al. [61]	Muffin (177°C, 48 min)	Egg	Lysozyme	FESNFNTQATNR	Not provided
				NTDGSTDYGILQINSR	
			Ovalbumin	ELINSWVESQTNGIIR	
				GGLEPINFQTAADQAR	
				HIATNAVLFFGR	
		Milk	αS1-casein	FFVAPFPEVFGK	
				HQGLPQEVLNENLLR	
				YLGYLEQLLR	
			β-lactoglobulin	LSFNPTQLEEQCHI	
				TPEVDDEALEK	
				VLVLDTDYK	

Authors	Matrix	Allergen	Protein	Peptide	Fragments
		Peanut	Ara h1	GTGNLELVAVR	
				NNPFYFPSR	
			Ara h2	CCNELNEFENNQR	
				CMCEALQQIMENQSDR	
				NLPQQCGLR	
			Ara h3	FNLAGNHEQEFLR	
				SPDIYNPQAGSLK	
				WLGLSAEYGNLYR	
Gomaa et al. 2014 [62]	Cookie (177°C, 12 min)	Milk	αS1-casein	HQGLPQEVLNENLLR	best transitions not selected
			αS2-casein	NAVPITPTLNR	
				LNFLK	
				ALNEINQFYQK	
			κ-casein	YIPIQYVLSR	
		Soy	Glycinin G1 precursor	HNIGQTSSPDIYNPQAGSVTTATSLDFPALSWLR	
				TNDTPMIGTLAGANSLLNALPEEVIQHTFNLK	
				VLIVPQNFVVAAR	
				HQQEEENEGGSILSGFTLEFLEHAFSVDK	
				EGDLIAVP...DQMPR	
			Glycinin G2 precursor	TNDRPSIGNLAGANSLLNALPEEVIQHTFNLK	
				QNIGQNSSPDIYNPQAGSITTATSLDFPALWLLK	
			Beta conglycinin alpha chain precursor	DLDIFLSIVDMNEGALLLPHFNSK	
				AIVILVINEGDANIELVGLK	
		Wheat	Alpha amylase trypsin inhibitor	YFIALPVPSQPVDPR	
				LLVAPGQCNLATIHNVR	
				LTAASITAVCR	
				LPIVVDASGDGAYVCK	
				SGNVGESGLIDLPGCPR	
				EMQWDFVR	
				DYVLQQTCGTFTPGSK	

Table 2b. List of target marker peptides used to detect several allergens in sauce, ice cream, chocolate, cookies and muffins [60–62].

lenge for laboratories is to achieve this sensitivity with processed foodstuffs. To reach this sensitivity, two factors must be considered: instrument sensitivity and optimization of sample preparation. The different strategies used to evaluate sensitivity are described below.

Instrument sensitivity: No comparison of the sensitivities of different instruments with the same peptide extract has yet been published for allergen analysis, although the sensitivity of the instrument is crucial to the sensitivity of the method, as in the case of other contaminants. One should bear in mind, however, that the most sensitive research-dedicated instrument might not be the best choice for routine analysis (automated injection and short analytical run).

Extraction and purification of proteins: The ideal sample preparation protocol should allow extraction of 100% of the target compounds, the final extract used for MS analysis being as pure as possible. Yet, the preparation of samples for food allergen analysis is difficult, because it should be applicable to a very broad range of food matrices and because the extractability of proteins might be altered in a processed food [63]. In addition, several modifications can occur, e.g. asparagine deamination, the Maillard reaction and several reactions of lysine. Such modifications cause a mass shift of tryptic peptides, resulting in non-recognition of several peptides by mass spectrometry [64–66]. To improve protein extraction, different parameters can be optimized: the composition of extraction buffers, the temperature, the sample-to-buffer ratio and the presence of detergents. Furthermore, the purification step is as important as extraction in order to concentrate proteins in and eliminate interferences from the supernatant. Purification usually involves solid phase extraction (SPE), protein precipitation, ultrafiltration and size exclusion chromatography (SEC), among others. Optimizing extraction and purification is a key step in developing sensitive methods for the detection of allergens by mass spectrometry (**Table 3**).

Determining the sensitivity: The sensitivity of food allergen analysis can be determined on spiked samples (obtained by incorporating extracted proteins into a matrix after processing), fortified samples (obtained by incorporating raw ingredients into a matrix after processing) or processed samples (obtained by incorporating raw ingredients into a matrix before processing). For spiked and fortified samples ('non-processed samples'), examples of the limit of quantification (LOQ) reached are 0.1 mg milk protein, 0.3 mg egg protein and 2 mg soy protein per kg cookies [67] and 0.1–1.3 mg tree nuts per kg biscuit [68]. Although these studies demonstrate the sensitivity of mass spectrometry, the real challenge is to reach this sensitivity in thermally processed samples. Important improvements have been made over the last 5 years in the detection of allergens in processed samples. Recently, developed methods allow reaching an LOQ near or below the VITAL threshold (**Table 1**), e.g. 0.5 mg for milk protein, 3.4 mg egg protein, 5 mg soy protein and 2.5 mg peanut protein per kg incurred cookie (180°C, 18 min, with SPE purification) [60]. In another study, the LOQs achieved were 30 mg egg (13.8 mg proteins), 20 mg milk (7.2 mg proteins), 19 mg soy (6.8 mg proteins), 20 mg hazelnut (3 mg proteins) and 40 mg peanut (10 mg proteins) per kg incurred cookie (200°C, 12 min, with SEC purification) [56].

As described above, the sensitivity reached for processed samples is lower than that obtained with spiked or fortified samples. The same applies to ELISAs, which can show up to 100-fold lower sensitivity when applied to processed food than when applied to raw food, as demonstrated by the poor performance of several ELISAs for egg detection in cookies after processing. In 2010, Dumont et al. showed that one ELISA kit was not even able to detect 1000 mg egg powder per kg baked cookie, and four others strongly underestimated the amount of egg in

Authors	Allergen	Matrix	Extraction	Purification	Digestion	Instrument	Sensitivity
Heick et al. (2010) [55]	Milk, egg, soy, peanut, hazelnut, walnut, almond	Bread (200°C, 60 min)	2 g/20 ml	Ultrafiltration (Amilcon Ultra 15 mL, 5 kDa molecular weight cut-off) (Millipore)	Dilution: 1 mg of proteins by ml with NH4HCO3 (100 mM)	LC: 1200 HPLC (Agilent)	LOD (S/N>3)
			Buffer: TRIS-HCl pH 8.2		Aliquot: 100 µl	Column: Xbridge C18 3.5 µm (2.1×150 mm) (Waters)	5 mg of soluble milk proteins by kg
			Agitation: 60°C for 3h		Reduction: 50 µl DTT (200 mM), 45 min	MS: API 4000QTrap (MDS Sciex)	42 mg of soluble egg proteins by kg
					Alkylation: 40 µl IA (1 M), 45 min in the dark		24 mg of soluble soy proteins by kg
					20 µl DTT (200 mM) + 50 µl NH4HCO3 (100 mM)		11 mg of soluble peanut proteins by kg
					Digestion: 10 µl trypsin (1 µg/µl) 12 h - 37°C		5 mg of soluble hazelnut proteins by kg
					2 µl formic acid		70 mg of soluble walnut proteins by kg
							3 mg of soluble almond proteins by kg
Pilolli et al. [56]	milk, egg,soy,peanut, hazelnut	Cookie (200°C, 12 min)	2.5 g/50 ml	1.2 µm acetate cellulose membrane, Size exclusion column (SEC) (G25 Sephadex column)	Elution SEC: 3.5 ml NH4HCO3 (50 mM)	LC: -	LOD (S/N>3)
			Buffer: 20 mM TRIS-HCl pH 8.2		Aliquot: 300 µl	Column: Aeris Peptide XB-C18 (150 × 2.1 mm) (Phenomenex)	7 mg of milk by kg
					Protein denaturation: 15 min at 95°C	MS: Dual pressure Linear Ion Trap Spectrometer Velos Pro (Thermo Fisher Scientic)	9 mg of egg by kg
			Ultrasound: 30 min		Reduction: 15 µl of 50 mM DTT 30 min at 60°C		6 mg of soy by kg
					Alkylation: 30 µl of 100 mM IAA 30 min in the dark at room temperature		13 mg of peanut by kg

Authors	Allergen	Matrix	Extraction	Purification	Digestion	Instrument	Sensitivity
					Digestion:4 μl trypsin (1 μg/μl) 14h		7 mg of hazelnut by kg
					Acidification: 1M HCl		
					Filtration: 0.2 μm		
Lamberti et al. [57]	Milk	Cookie (180°C, 10 min)	10 mg /200 μl	Protein precipitation methanol/ chloroform	Pellet + 50 μl of 0.025M NH4HCO3 pH 8.0 RT	LC: HP 1100 HPLC (Agilent)	LOD: 1.3 mg of milk proteins per kg
			Buffer: NH4HCO3 / (NH4)2CO3 +1 % SDS buffer, pH 8.2		3 μl of trypisn (75 ng/μl) 37°C, 90 min	Column: ACE C18 300A (250 mm × 1 mm)	LOQ: 4 mg of milk proteins per kg
			Agitation: 20 min, 60°C		5 μl of 5% formic acid	MS: XCT-Plus Ion trap mass spectrometer (Agilent)	
Pedreschi et al. [58]	Peanut	Cookie (180°C, 16 min)	Buffer: 20 mM TRIS - 150 mM NaCl, pH 7.4	GE Healthcare kit	50 μg of protein / 50 μl of Rapigest in a 50 mM ammonium bicarbonate buffer	LC: nano Acquity UPLC (Waters)	>10 mg of peanut per kg
			Ultrasound: 4°C, 20 min	Cut-off filtration 3000 MWCO	2.5 μl of 50 mM DTT 30 min, 60°C	Column: nano Acquity BEH130 C18 1.7 μm (75 μm × 100 mm)	
					5 μl 100 mM IAA 30 min-dark	Column: nano Acquity UPLC Trap SymC18 5 μm (180 μm × 20 mm)	
					1 μl of 1μg/μm of trypsin 5h-37°C	MS: Q-Tof Ultima Global (Waters)	

Table 3a. Mass-spectrometry-based methods (extraction, purification, digestion, and analysis) for detecting allergens in processed food products [55–58].

Author	Allergens	Matrices	Extraction	Purification	Digestion	Instrument	Sensitivity
Huschek et al. [59]	Soy, sesame, lupin	Wheat, cookie (190°C, 13 min), bread (220°C, 30 min)	1 g	SPE cardridge (LiChrolut RP-18 Merck Millipore)	Alkylation: IAA 20 min at 50°C	LC: Nexera XR UHPLC (Shimadzu)	LOQ (S/N > 10)
			Buffer: 100 mM NH4HCO3, 4M urea 5 mM DTT pH 8.2		Digestion: Trypsin	Column: Aeris Peptide XB-C18 (100 × 2.1 mm, 1.7 µm) (Phenomenex)	10–20 mg of soy per kg
					formic acid 2%		10–50 mg of sesame per kg
			Agitation 30 min RT			MS: Qtrap 5500 MS/MS (Sciex)	10–50 mg of lupine per kg
Planque et al. [33, 60]	Milk, egg, soy, peanut	Tomato sauce (95°C, 45 min), cookie (180°C, 18 min), ice cream, chocolate	2 g / 20 ml	Sep-Pack tC18 6cc (Waters)	10 ml extract + 10 ml NH4HCO3 (200 mM)	LC: UPLC Acquity (Waters)	LOQ (S/N > 10)
			Buffer: 200 mM TRIS-HCl pH 9.2, 2M urea		Reduction: 1 ml DTT (400 mM), 45 min	Column: BEH130 (2.1 × 150 mm) (Waters)	0.5 mg of milk proteins by kg
					Alkylation: 2 ml IAA (500 mM), 45 min in the dark	MS: Xevo TQS (Waters)	3.4 mg of egg proteins by kg
			Agitation:30 min Ultrasound: 15 min		Digestion: Ratio protein:trypsin 1:20 16 h, 37°C		5 mg of soy proteins by kg
					300 µl formic acid 20%		2.5 mg of peanut proteins by kg
Parker et al. [61]	Milk, egg, peanut	Muffin (177°C, 48 min)	Buffer: 2 M urea, 50 mM TRIS Ph 8.0, 25 mM DTT	Microcentrifuge tubes	Filter-aided sample preparation (FASP) sample cocentration and digestion protocol	LC: nano Acquity UPLC (Waters)	/
				Amicon Ultra 0.5 ml	Reduction: 10 mM DTT	Column: nano Acquity BEH130 C18 1.7 µm (100 µm × 100 mm)	
			vortex: 5 min at 1400 rpm	Utracel-10 membrane	Alkylation:25 mM IAA	MS:6500 QTRAP (Sciex)	
			Ultrasound: 10 min at 4°C		Digestion: Ratio protein:trypsin 1:100 16 h -37°C		
					0.1% trifluoroacetic acid and 2% acetonitrile		

http://dx.doi.org/10.5772/intechopen.69361

Author	Allergens	Matrices	Extraction	Purification	Digestion	Instrument	Sensitivity
Gomaa et al. [62]	Milk, soy, wheat	Cookie (177°C, 12 min)	1 g/9 ml	OMIX C18/ tip (Varian)	Protein extract: 100 μl at 2 mg/ml	LC: nano Acquity UPLC (Waters)	10 mg of casein per kg
			Buffer: 50 mM NH4HCO3		Reduction: 1μl of DTT (0.5 M) 56°C, 20 min	Column: nano Acquity BEH130 C18 1.7 μm (75 μm × 100 mm)	10 mg of soy proteins per kg
					Alkylation: 2.7 μl IAA (0.55 M, 15 min)	nano Acquity UPLC Trap SymC18 5 μm (180 μm × 20 mm)	100 mg of gluten per kg
					Digestion: ratio enzyme:subtrate 1:20 3h-37°C	MS: Q-Tof Synapt MS (Waters)	
					5 μl trifluoroacetic acid (2.5%)		

Table 3b. Mass-spectrometry-based methods (extraction, purification, digestion, and analysis) for detecting allergens in processed chocolate, sauce, ice cream, muffins and cookies [59–62].

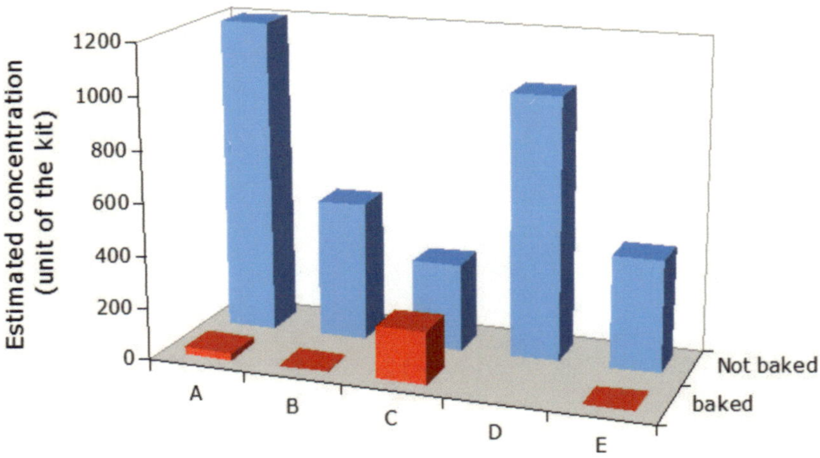

Figure 4. Analytical results for 1000 mg spray-dried whole egg powder (National Institute of Standards and Technology RM 8445) per kg incurred cookies, obtained with the different enzyme-linked immunosorbent assay test kits for egg detection (A–E) (from Ref. [69]).

the samples (**Figure 4** of Ref. [69]). While mass spectrometry and ELISAs show comparable sensitivities when applied to unbaked products, mass spectrometry seems to be the method of choice for the analysis of allergens in baked food products.

3. Quantifying food allergens

Detecting hidden allergens in food products is essential to protecting the food-allergic population. For full transparency of allergen labelling, laboratories should also be able to quantify allergens in order to help food manufacturers manage cross-contamination during food production [70]. However, significant signal suppressions have been observed in various food matrices, and the level of suppression depends on the matrix considered. In one study, for example, high-protein-content food products showed greater suppression of the peptide signal than ones with a low protein content: the determined LOQ values were 20 mg skim milk powder per kg for high-protein foods and 5 mg skim milk powder per kg for low-protein foods [71]. The food protein content is not the only parameter to be considered in relation to suppression of the peptide signal obtained by mass spectrometry: factors such as the type of process, the fat content and the presence of tannins also have an important influence on food allergen detection and must be taken into account.

While detecting allergens in various food products is difficult, quantifying them is even worse. In recent years, mass spectrometry techniques have been used for quantitation in proteomic analysis. Two approaches have emerged as the most relevant for food allergen quantification: label-free quantification and the use of stable-isotope-labelled peptides or proteins [70, 72, 73]. The two strategies are compared in **Table 4** (target peptides, internal standards and calibration curves) and discussed in relation to the AOAC guideline 2016.002 method performance requirements for the quantification of allergens in food products, specifying a recovery between 60 and 120% and intra-day and inter-day coefficients of variation lower than 20 and 30%, respectively [74] (**Table 5**).

http://dx.doi.org/10.5772/intechopen.69361

Authors	Matrix	Allergen	Protein	Peptide	Mass spectrometer	Internal standard	Calibration curve
Careri et al. [76]	Rice crispy/ chocolate snacks	Peanut	Ara h2	CCNELNEFENNQR	Q-TOF Micro (Waters)	No internal standard	Rice crispy/ chocolate snacks were spiked with peanut proteins
				CMCEALQQIMENQSDR			
			Ara h3/4	AHVQVVDSNGDR			
				SPDIYNPQAGSLK			
Monaci et al. [75]	Fruit juices	Milk	α-lactalbumin	/	Ultima triple quadrupole mass spectrometer (Waters)	No internal standard	Fruit juices were spiked with milk proteins
			β-lactoglobulin A				
			β-lactoglobulin B				
Korte et al. [88]	Bread matrix, ice cream, chocolate, muesli with fruit and berry	Almond	Pru du 6.0101	GNLDFVQPPR	QTRAP 6500 (Sciex)	No internal standard	Matrices were spiked with allergen proteins
			Pru du 6.0201	VQGQLDFVSPFSR			
				ALPDEVLQNAFR			
		Cashew	Ana o2	ADIYTPEVGR			
				EGQMLVVPQNFAVVK			
				LTTLNSLNLPILK			
		Hazelnut	Cor a 9	LNALEPTNR			
				VQVVDDNGNTVFDDELR			
				QGQVLTIPQNFAVAK			
		Peanut	Ara h3	FNLAGNHEQEFLR			
				WLGLSAEYGNLYR			
				TANDLNLLILR			

Authors	Matrix	Allergen	Protein	Peptide	Mass spectrometer	Internal standard	Calibration curve
		Pistachio	Pis v 5	AMISPLAGSTSVLR			
				ITSLNSLNLPILK			
				GFESEEESEYER			
		Walnut	Jug r 2	FFDQQEQR			
				ATLTLVSQETR			
			Jug r4	ALPEEVLATAFQIPR			
Mattarozzi et al. [77]	Pasta, biscuit	Lupin	β-conglutin	IVEFQSKPNTLILPK	LTQ XL linear ion trap (Thermo)	No internal standard	Pasta and biscuits were fortified with lupin proteins
Zhang et al. [78]	Infant formulas and whey proteins	Milk	α-lactalbumin	VGINYWLAHK	Xevo TQ triple quadrupole (Waters)	KILDKVGINNYWLAHKALCSE	Matrices were spiked with synthetic peptide VGINYWLAHK
Posada-Ayala et al. [79]	Sauces and salty biscuit	Mustard	Sin a1	ACQQWLHK	6460 triple quadrupole (Agilent technologies)	Purified protein Sin a 1	Standard addition of mustard in sauces and salty biscuits
				IYQTATHLPK			
				EFQQAQHLR			

Table 4a. Quantification of food allergens in different food products by mass spectrometry using label-free quantification with an (1) external calibration curve [75–79, 88], (2) unlabelled modified synthetic peptide [78], and (3) standard addition [79].

Authors	Matrix	Allergen	Protein	Peptide	Mass spectrometer	Internal standard	Calibration curve
Newsome and Scholl [82]	Cookie (180°C, 16 min)	Milk	α-s1 casein	HQGLPQEVLNENLLR	Hybrid triple-quadrupole 4000 QTRAP (AB Sciex)	HQGLPQEVLNENLLR[13C, 15N]	Cookies were spiked with isotope labelled peptides
				YLGYLEQLLR		YLGYLEQLLR[13C6, 15N]	
				FFVAPFPEVFGK		FFVAPFPEVF[13C6, 15N]GK	
						15N-α-s1 casein	
Parker et al. [61]	Cereal bar (177°C, 30 min) Muffin (177°C, 48 min)	Egg	Lysozyme	NTDGSTDYGILQINSR	6500 Qtrap (AB Sciex)	Heavy isotope [13C, 15N] labelled peptides / labelled amino acid: R or K	Cereal and muffin were spiked with isotope labelled peptides
			Ovalbumin	GGLEPINFQTAADQAR			
		Milk	α-s1 casein	YLGYLEQLLR			
			β-lactoglobulin	LSFNPTQLEEQCHI			
		Peanut	Ara h1	NNPFYFPSR			
			Ara h2	NLPQQCGLR			
			Ara h3	SPDIYNPQAGSLK			
Huschek et al. [59]	Wheat, cookies (190°C, 13 min), soft bread (220°C-	Soy	Gly m6	VFDGELQEGR	QTRAP 5500 (Sciex)	VFDGELQEGR[13C6, 15N4]	Wheat and cookies were spiked with allergen proteins
		Sesame	Ses i6	ISGAQPSLR		ISGAQPSLR[13C6, 15N4]	
		Lupin	β-conglutin	LLGFGINADENQR		LLGFGINADENQR[13C6, 15N4]	
Lutter et al. (2011) [71]	Baby food soy-based formula, infant cereals, breakfast cereals, rince water	Milk	β-casein	AVPYPQR	6460 triple quadrupole (Agilent technologies)	AVPYPQR [13C6, 15N4]	0.1% formic acid were spiked with proteins
			α-s2 casein	ALNEINQFYQK		ALNEINQFYQK[13C6, 15N2]	
			α-s2 casein	FALPQYLK		FALPQYLK[13C6, 15N2]	
			κ-casein	YIPIQYVLSR		YIPIQYVLSR[13C6, 15N2]	
			β-lactoglobulin	TPEVDDEALEK		TPEVDDEALEK[13C6, 15N2]	
				VLVLDTDYK		VLVLDTDYK[13C6, 15N4]	
Monaci et al. [75]	White wine	Milk	α-s1 casein	FFVAPFPEVFGK	Extractive ESI Orbitrap (Thermo Electron)	FFV[15N]APFPEV[15N]FGK	White wine were spiked with milk and egg proteins
		Egg	Ovalbumin	LTEWTSSNVMEER		LTEWTSSNV[15N]MEER	

Authors	Matrix	Allergen	Protein	Peptide	Mass spectrometer	Internal standard	Calibration curve
Yi-Shun et al. (2017) [84]	Beer, wine, chips, flour, cookies…	Gluten	α-glyadin γ-Hordein	LWQIPEQSR QQCCQQLANINEQSR	6490 triple quad (Agilent)	LWQIPEQSR[13C, 15N] QQCCQQLANINEQSR [13C, 15N]	Matrices were spiked with gluten proteins
Ippoushi et al. [89]	Sweet cherry fruit	Cherry	Pru av2	TGCCAMSTDASGK	Xevo TQD Zspray ion source (Waters)	TGCCAMSTDASGK[13C6,15N2]	Sweet cherry fruit were spiekd with isotope labelled peptides
Rahman et al. (2012) [90]	/	Shrimp	Tropomyosine Arginine kinase	SEEEVFGLQK QQLVDDHFLFVSGDR	Micro mass Quattro Ultima (Waters)	SEEEV[D8]VFGLQK QQLV[D8]VDDHFLFV[D8]SGDR	Solvent were spiked with shrimp proteins
Chen et al. (2014) [83]	Baked food (170°C, 25 min)	Milk	β-casein	VLPVPQR	TOF-MS Synapt G2 HDMS (Waters)	VL[13C6, 15N]PV[13C5, 15N]PQK (IS1) QSVLSLSQSKVL[13C6, 15N]PV[13C5, 15N]PQKAVPYPQRQ (IS2) Human β-casein (IS3)	Solvent were spiked with milk proteins

Table 4b. Quantification of food allergens in different food products by mass spectrometry using stable isotope labelling quantification with an (1) isotope-labelled protein [82], (2) isotope-labelled peptide [59, 61, 71, 75, 84, 89, 90] or (3) long isotope-labelled peptide [83].

Parameter	Target allergen			
	Whole egg	Milk	Peanut	Hazelnut
Analytical range, ppm	10–1000	10–1000	10–1000	10–1000
MLQ, ppm	≤5	≤10	≤10	≤10
MDL, ppm	≤1.65	≤3	≤3	≤3
Recovery %	60–120	60–120	60–120	60–120
RSD_r %	≤20	≤20	≤20	≤20
RSD_R %	≤30	≤30	≤30	≤30
Reported as ppm of the target allergen in food commodity i.e. 25 ppm of 'whole egg' in cookies.				

Table 5. Method performance requirements from the AOAC guideline SMPR 2016.002 for egg, milk, peanut and hazelnut allergens in terms of analytical range, method quantification limit, recovery and intra-day and inter-day coefficients of variation (table from Paez et al. [74]).

3.1. Label-free quantification

The label-free quantification strategy is based on comparing the peptide signal intensities of different samples (**Table 4a**). Three label-free quantification possibilities are described below.

External calibration: Monaci et al. used this approach to quantify milk proteins in fruit juice. Using a calibration curve obtained by spiking fruit juice with extracted milk proteins, they found recoveries between 68 and 79% [75]. This strategy was also used to quantify peanut proteins in rice crispy/chocolate snacks [76]. A significant suppression effect, ranging from 30 to 50%, was observed for the Ara h2 peptide signal, while suppression of the Ara h3/4 peptide signal was less than 10%. A more recent study by Mattarozzi et al. obtained recoveries between 95 and 118% for lupin β-conglutin peptide in spiked biscuits [77]. Although less expensive than other approaches, this approach requires a calibration curve for each matrix.

Modified synthetic peptide approach: Zhang et al. introduced an internal standard peptide (KILDKVGINNYWLAHKALCSE) with an added asparagine residue (N) in the β-casein peptide VGINYWLAHK. They obtained recoveries between 98.8 and 100.6% [78]. The use of an internal standard allows better recovery, but adding an amino acid can change the retention time and modify the ionization of target peptides.

Standard addition: This label-free quantification strategy consists in adding standards to the matrices. It was used by Posada-Ayala et al. for the quantification of commercial food products [79]. This approach consists in adding different known quantities of extracted allergen proteins directly to the sample to be analysed before digestion and in quantifying the target allergens with the resulting calibration curve. The recovery was not specified, but this approach allows correcting at least for digestion and matrix effects. However, the theoretical level of contamination in the samples must be known in order to adapt the quantities of standards to be added.

3.2. Stable isotope labelling quantification

This strategy is based on the use of isotope-labelled (^{13}C-, ^{15}N-, D-labelled) peptides or proteins [80] (**Table 4b**). It is recommend to use a 6-Da mass difference with respect to the amino acid for doubly charged precursors and an 8–10-Da mass difference for triply charged precursors [52]. Although more expensive than the strategies described above, this approach has the advantage that the unlabelled and isotope-labelled peptides show similar ionization and similar mass spectrometry response signals. For allergen quantification, three kinds of isotope-labelled standards exist [81]: proteins [82], concatemers [83] (or long isotope-labelled peptides) and Aqua peptides [61, 71, 75, 84] (isotope-labelled peptides) (**Figure 5**).

Isotope-labelled proteins: The principle of this approach is to add a labelled protein to the sample before extraction. Newsome et al. studied the recovery of the milk allergen α-S1 casein in baked cookies using a labelled internal α-S1 casein, and obtained recoveries ranging from 60 to 80% [82]. Use of an internal standard allows correcting for the matrix effect and for effects linked to different steps in the sample preparation protocol (protein extraction and enzymatic digestion). It thus allows accurate determination of the recovery and precision for processed samples. This 'gold standard' approach is really expensive, however, making its use unrealistic for the vast majority of routine laboratories.

Isotope-labelled peptides: The principle is to add labelled peptides to the sample after digestion and before the purification steps. This approach is less expensive than the use of isotope-labelled proteins, and synthetic labelled peptides can easily be commercially obtained. Huschek et al. used isotope-labelled peptides to quantify soy, lupin and sesame allergens [59]. They determined the recovery of their method by spiking wheat, cookie and bread with the labelled peptides and obtained results between 69.4 and 112.9%. One could argue, however, that very similar matrices were used in this study (wheat-based products) and that this type of study should be extended to other matrices in order to validate the ability of the isotope-labelled peptide to correct for matrix effects.

Lutter et al. quantified milk proteins in baby food, infant cereals, breakfast cereals and rinsing water, using a calibration curve obtained by spiking 0.1% formic acid with milk protein. The estimated recovery rates were between 16 and 66% [71] Lutter et al. In this study, the isotope-labelled peptides were used to correct for effects related to different steps of the analysis. While using a single calibration curve can be useful in the routine laboratory context, the relatively low recoveries obtained in this study reveal the inability of an isotope-labelled peptide to correct for sample-preparation-related effects. We have compared the areas of milk, egg, peanut and soy peptide peaks for three matrices with and without isotope labelled peptides. Our results clearly show that an isotope-labelled peptide is able to correct for matrix effects but not for effects linked to the extraction and digestion steps [85] planque et al.

Isotope-labelled concatemers/long isotope-labelled peptides: The isotope-labelled concatemer used in this technique is a chimeric protein containing all the labelled target peptides.

http://dx.doi.org/10.5772/intechopen.69361

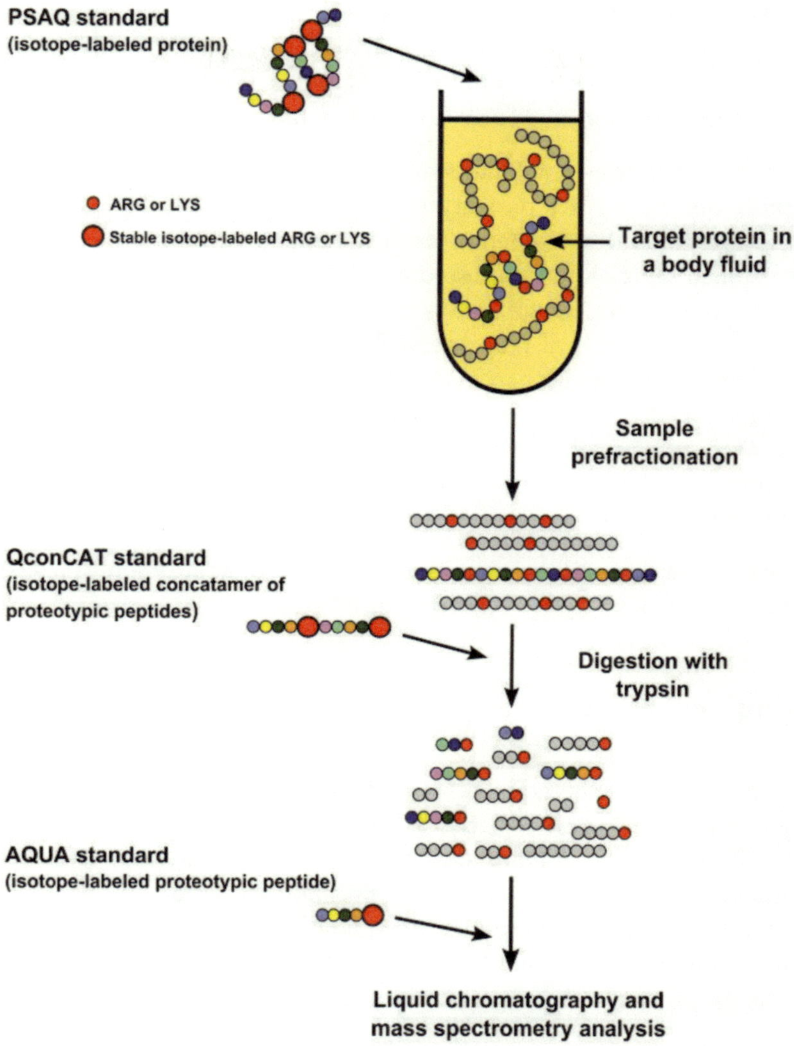

Figure 5. Three types of internal standards are used for the quantification of proteins by mass spectrometry (1) isotope-labelled protein (2) Isotope-labelled concatemers or long isotope-labelled peptides (3) isotope-labelled peptide (from Ref. [81]).

This internal standard is added to the sample before enzymatic digestion. The advantage of this method is that a single concatemer can contain peptides belonging to different proteins or allergens. This strategy has been used in proteomics, but it is not yet used for food allergen quantification [86]. An emerging alternative to use of a concatemer is use of a so-called 'long isotope-labelled peptide'. Chen et al. compared the use of three types of internal standard: human β-casein, isotope-labelled peptide VL [$^{13}C_6$, ^{15}N] PV[$^{13}C_5$, ^{15}N]PQK and a long isotope-labelled peptide QSVLSLSQSKVL[$^{13}C_6$,^{15}N] PV[$^{13}C_5$,^{15}N]PQKAVPYPQRQ [83]. The long isotope-labelled peptide provided better recovery, due to correction for digestion-step-related effects. The recovery based on spiked materials was between 98.8 and 106.7%. In 2016, it was shown that long isotope-labelled peptides allow recoveries of 97.2–102.5% for α-lactalbumin and 99.5–100.3% for β-casein in the quantification of human milk [87]. This strategy is a good compromise between isotope-labelled proteins and peptides. It allows correcting both for the matrix effect and for digestion-step effects, unlike the use of isotope-labelled peptides.

In conclusion, these studies show that using an isotope-labelled protein or a long isotope-labelled peptide provides better recovery than the isotope-labelled peptide approach. As explained below in the section devoted to result validation, the recovery must be determined with allergen-spiked samples and processed matrices in order to meet AOAC specifications. Published methods, however, do not always meet the AOAC requirements, even with spiked samples. For instance, Careri et al. [76] observed a suppression effect between 30 and 50% for the Ara h2 peptide signal, and Monaci et al. [75] obtained recoveries ranging from 68 to 79% for α-lactalbumin and β lactoglobulin. Altogether, these works show that internal standards are needed for the quantification of allergens in food matrices. Currently, furthermore, the use of a calibration curve for each type of sample is the best way to respect the AOAC guideline requiring a recovery between 60 and 120%.

Future studies should thus still be done to improve the quantification of allergens from a single calibration curve with a good recovery.

4. Validating food allergen methods

While mass spectrometry methods are increasingly sensitive, there remains room for improvement. Furthermore, there subsist obstacles to the harmonization of allergen detection methods in food laboratories [85]. In April 2016, the AOAC SMPR 2016.002 guideline 'Standard method requirements for the detection and quantification of selected food allergens' was published. This guideline is the first to specify target limits for sensitivity and range of linearity, target matrices and reference materials for the analysis of allergens (egg, milk, peanut and hazelnut) in food matrices by mass spectrometry (**Table 5**).

To obtain comparable results among laboratories, it is crucial to adopt validation guidelines. The AOAC guideline, however, is not sufficiently detailed, and each laboratory tends to apply its own rules. In what follows, we compare this guideline with published methods in terms of sensitivity, range of linearity, recovery and precision.

Sensitivity: In the AOAC guideline, the method quantitation limit (MQL) is defined as MQL = average (blank) + 10 x s_0 (blank). Laboratories, however, often use other strategies to determine the limit of quantification (LOQ), such as determining a signal-to-noise (S/N) ratio which should be higher than 10 [56, 60] or estimating an LOD and an LOQ as 3s/slope and 10s/slope, respectively, where s is the standard deviation of the blank signal (n = 10) [57]. On the other hand, the sensitivity can differ from one matrix to another. For example, in a study where cookie, ice cream and sauce were spiked with 0.5 mg milk proteins per kg, the observed S/N ratio was 26 for the cookie matrix, 83 for ice cream and 228 for sauce [85]. This also highlights the importance of a 'fit-for-purpose' description of an analytical method. Moreover, the sensitivities of developed methods should be determined on the same reference materials (MoniQa, LGC) to ensure (1) their capacity to reach the sensitivity set by the AOAC guideline and (2) an appropriate comparison of method performances.

Linearity: The range of linearity is set as 0.001 to 0.1% allergen contamination (10 mg to 1000 mg) of allergenic ingredients per kg) and thus does not always include the MQL (e. g. an MLQ_{egg} of 5 mg per kg). In the case of high-sensitivity methods, the coefficient of regression is determined using a lower range of concentrations [57, 71].

Recovery: Recovery must range from 60 to 120%. Such recovery values are hard to reach for the detection of allergens in processed samples, and recovery can only be determined by spiking food matrices with allergens. Focusing on egg, milk and peanut in spiked and incurred muffin and cereal bars, Parker et al. constructed calibration curves by spiking the matrices with allergen proteins [61]. In the case of spiked muffin, the determined recovery was 98.6% for egg peptide (GGLEPINFQTAADQAR), 87.7% for milk peptide (YLGYLEQLLR) and 100.2% for peanut peptide (SPDIYNPQAGSLK). When the muffins were baked for 48 min at 177°C, the recoveries were dramatically lower: respectively 45.2%, 75.2% and 70.2%.

Inter- and intra-day coefficients of variation: According to AOAC SPMR, three unknown samples should be analyzed at least seven times to determine the reproducibility of the method. Lamberti et al. determined an intra-day coefficient of variation between 5 and 20% by performing three independent extractions at two different concentrations and three injections per extract [57].

Guidelines for the validation of mass-spectrometry-based methods for allergen analysis should be more precise, like the guidelines 2002/657/EC 'Validation of residues in products of animal origin' and SANCO/12574/2013 'Residues in products of animal origin method validation procedures for pesticide residues analysis in food and feed'. In SMPR 2016.002, several details are missing:

- The number of target peptides that a method should include to confirm the presence of an allergen, as well as fragment ion number and/or type.
- Criteria for the relative retention time, the ion ratio and the specificity of the method (blast, analysis of different blank and matrices), the level of spiking for determining precision and accuracy (for example, the LOQ, action limit and upper limit).

5. Conclusion

The major increase of the allergic population has prompted the development of numerous allergen detection methods. Over the past few years, improvements in the detection of allergens by mass spectrometry have been impressive, allowing detection of processed allergens with high sensitivity (a few mg of proteins per kg of food). Optimization of extraction and purification steps has notably played a key role in the improvement of analytical methods. Allergen quantification is performed mainly with labelled internal standards.

The best approach involves the use of labelled proteins, allowing correction for effects occurring throughout the sample preparation protocol. The high cost of labelled proteins, however, has promoted the use of other strategies, such as methods based on long isotope-labelled peptides and standard addition of allergens.

The validation of qualitative and quantitative MS-based methods for routine detection of allergens is still very recent. The AOAC guideline is a first step towards the development of methods that will allow procedure harmonization, making it possible to compare results between laboratories. These methods should be both improved and extended to other allergens in order to demonstrate their validity and robustness.

Author details

Mélanie Planque[1,2], Thierry Arnould[2] and Nathalie Gillard[1]*

*Address all correspondence to: n.gillard@cergroupe.be

1 Health Department, CER Groupe, Marloie, Belgium

2 Laboratory of Biochemistry and Cell Biology (URBC), Namur Research Institute for Life Sciences (NARILIS), University of Namur, Namur, Belgium

References

[1] Wang J, Sampson HA, Rona R, Branum A, Lukacs S, Sicherer S, et al. Food allergy. Journal of Clinical Investigation [Internet]. American Society for Clinical Investigation. 2011;**121**(3):827-835. Available from: http://www.jci.org/articles/view/45434 [Accessed: 10 June 2016]

[2] Manea I, Ailenei E, Deleanu D. Overview of food allergy diagnosis. Clujul medical (1957) [Internet]. 2016;**89**(1):5-10. Available from: http://www.pubmedcentral.nih.gov/articlerender.fcgi?artid=4777468&tool=pmcentrez&rendertype=abstract [Accessed: 9 April 2016]

[3] Tam JS. Cutaneous manifestation of food allergy. Immunology and Allergy Clinics of North America [Internet]. 2017;**37**(1):217-231. Available from: http://linkinghub.elsevier.com/retrieve/pii/S0889856116300765 [Accessed: 23 March 2017]

[4] Sampson HA. Update on food allergy☆. Journal of Allergy and Clinical Immunology [Internet]. 2004;**113**(5):805-819. Available from: http://www.ncbi.nlm.nih.gov/pubmed/15131561 [Accessed: 23 March 2017]

[5] Ho MH-K, Wong WH-S, Chang C. Clinical spectrum of food allergies: A comprehensive review. Clinical Reviews in Allergy & Immunology [Internet]. USA: Springer. 2014;**46**(3):225-240. Available from: http://link.springer.com/10.1007/s12016-012-8339-6 [Accessed: 10 June 2016]

[6] Cianferoni A, Muraro A. Food-induced anaphylaxis. Immunology and Allergy Clinics of North America [Internet]. NIH Public Access. 2012;**32**(1):165-195. Available from: http://www.ncbi.nlm.nih.gov/pubmed/22244239 [Accessed: 7 March 2017]

[7] Sindher S, Fleischer DM, Spergel JM. Advances in the treatment of food allergy. Immunology and Allergy Clinics of North America [Internet]. 2016;**36**(1):39-54. Available from: http://www.ncbi.nlm.nih.gov/pubmed/26617226 [Accessed: 15 March 2017]

[8] Tordesillas L, Mondoulet L, Blazquez AB, Benhamou P-H, Sampson HA, Berin MC. Epicutaneous immunotherapy induces gastrointestinal LAP+ regulatory T cells and prevents food-induced anaphylaxis. Journal of Allergy and Clinical Immunology [Internet]. 2017;**139**(1):189-201.e4. Available from: http://www.ncbi.nlm.nih.gov/pubmed/27417020 [Accessed: 7 March 2017]

[9] Ravid NL, Annunziato RA, Ambrose MA, Chuang K, Mullarkey C, Sicherer SH, et al. Mental health and quality-of-life concerns related to the burden of food allergy. Psychiatric Clinics of North America [Internet]. 2015;**38**(1):77-89. Available from: http://linkinghub.elsevier.com/retrieve/pii/S0193953X14001014 [Accessed: 7 March 2017]

[10] King RM, Knibb RC, Hourihane JO. Impact of peanut allergy on quality of life, stress and anxiety in the family. Allergy [Internet]. 2009;**64**(3):461-468. Available from: http://www.ncbi.nlm.nih.gov/pubmed/19076542 [Accessed: 26 April 2016]

[11] Gendel SM. Comparison of international food allergen labeling regulations. Regulatory Toxicology and Pharmacology. 2012;**63**:279-285

[12] Regulation (EU) No 1169/2011 of the European parliament and of the council of 25 October 2011. 2011

[13] Spanjersberg MQI, Knulst AC, Kruizinga AG, Van Duijn G, Houben GF. Concentrations of undeclared allergens in food products can reach levels that are relevant for public health. Food Additives & Contaminants: Part A [Internet]. Taylor & Francis Group. 2010;**27**(2):169-174. Available from: http://www.tandfonline.com/doi/abs/10.1080/19440040903317513 [Accessed: 30 September 2016]

[14] DZWOLAK, Waldemar. Assessment of food allergen management in small food facilities. Food Control, 2017;**73**:323-331

[15] Hefle SL, Taylor SL. Food allergy and the food industry. Current Allergy and Asthma Reports [Internet]. Current Medicine Group. 2004;**4**(1):55-59. Available from: http://link.springer.com/10.1007/s11882-004-0044-y [Accessed: 22 November 2016]

[16] WALKER, M. J., BURNS, D. T., ELLIOTT, C. T., et al. Is food allergen analysis flawed? Health and supply chain risks and a proposed framework to address urgent analytical needs. Analyst, 2016;**141**(1):24-35

[17] DunnGalvin A, Chan C-H, Crevel R, Grimshaw K, Poms R, Schnadt S, et al. Precautionary allergen labelling: Perspectives from key stakeholder groups. Allergy [Internet]. 2015;**70**(9):1039-1051. Available from: http://doi.wiley.com/10.1111/all.12614 [Accessed: 14 June 2016]

[18] Zurzolo GA, Mathai ML, Koplin JJ, Allen KJ. Precautionary allergen labelling following new labelling practice in Australia. Journal of Paediatrics and Child Health [Internet]. 2013;**49**(4):E306-310. Available from: http://doi.wiley.com/10.1111/jpc.12138 [Accessed: 22 November 2016]

[19] Pele M, Brohée M, Anklam E, Van Hengel AJ. Peanut and hazelnut traces in cookies and chocolates: Relationship between analytical results and declaration of food allergens on product labels. Food Additives and Contaminants [Internet]. 2007;**24**(12):1334-1344. Available from: http://www.ncbi.nlm.nih.gov/pubmed/17852393 [Accessed: 26 April 2016]

[20] Marchisotto MJ, Harada L, Blumenstock JA, Bilaver LA, Waserman S, Sicherer S, et al. Global perceptions of food allergy thresholds in 16 countries. Allergy [Internet]. 2016;**71**(8):1081-1085. Available from: htt://doi.wiley.com/10.1111/all.12933 [Accessed: 16 March 2017]

[21] BUCCHINI, Luca, GUZZON, Antonella, POMS, Roland, et al. Analysis and critical comparison of food allergen recalls from the European Union, USA, Canada, Hong Kong, Australia and New Zealand. Food Additives & Contaminants: Part A, 2016;**33**(5):760-771

[22] Gendel Sm, Zhu J. Analysis of U.S. food and drug administration food allergen recalls after Implementation of the food allergen labeling and consumer protection act. Journal of Food Protection [Internet]. 2013;**76**(11):1933-1938. Available from: http://www.ncbi.nlm.nih.gov/pubmed/24215698 [Accessed: 13 April 2017]

[23] U S Food and Drug Administration Home Page [Internet].. Available from: https://www.fda.gov/ [Accessed: 13 April 2017]

[24] The Rapid Alert System for Food and Feed https://ec.europa.eu/food/safety/rasff_en

[25] Bienvenue à l'Agence canadienne d'inspection des aliments - Agence canadienne d'inspection des aliments [Internet].. Available from: http://www.inspection.gc.ca/fra/1297964599443/1297965645317 [Accessed: 13 April 2017]

[26] Recalls | Product Safety Australia [Internet]. Available from: https://www.productsafety.gov.au/recalls?source=recalls [Accessed: 13 April 2017]

[27] VITAL ® Voluntary Incidental Trace Allergen Labelling | Allergen Bureau [Internet].. Available from: http://allergenbureau.net/vital/ [Accessed: 13 April 2017]

[28] Home | NVWA [Internet].. Available from: https://www.nvwa.nl/ [Accessed: 13 April 2017]

[29] Tolin S, Pasini G, Curioni A, Arrigoni G, Masi A, Mainente F, et al. Mass spectrometry detection of egg proteins in red wines treated with egg white. Food Control. 2012;**23**:87-94

[30] Weber D, Raymond P, Ben-Rejeb S, Lau B. Development of a liquid chromatography-tandem mass spectrometry method using capillary liquid chromatography and nano-electrospray ionization-quadrupole time-of-flight hybrid mass spectrometer for the

detection of milk allergens. Journal of Agricultural and Food Chemistry [Internet]. 2006;**54**(5):1604-1610. Available from: https://vpn.gw.ulg.ac.be/doi/abs/10.1021/,DanaInfo=pubs.acs.org+jf052464s [Accessed: 28 April 2016]

[31] Korte R, Lepski S, Brockmeyer J. Comprehensive peptide marker identification for the detection of multiple nut allergens using a non-targeted LC-HRMS multi-method. Analytical and Bioanalytical Chemistry [Internet]. 2016;**408**(12):3059-3069. Available from: http://www.ncbi.nlm.nih.gov/pubmed/26894760 [Accessed: 23 September 2016]

[32] Houston NL, Lee D-G, Stevenson SE, Ladics GS, Bannon GA, McClain S, et al. Quantitation of soybean allergens using tandem mass spectrometry. Journal of Proteome Research [Internet]. 2011;**10**(2):763-773. Available from: http://www.ncbi.nlm.nih.gov/pubmed/21141899 [Accessed: 27 March 2017]

[33] Planque M, Wallace A, Gillard N. [Application Note] Targeted and Sensitive Detection of Food Allergens in Complex and Processed Foodstuffs Using UPLC-MS/MS [APPLICATION NOTE]. 2016;1-6

[34] Taylor SL, Baumert JL, Kruizinga AG, Remington BC, Crevel RWR, Brooke-Taylor S, et al. Establishment of Reference Doses for residues of allergenic foods: Report of the vital expert panel. Food and Chemical Toxicology. 2014;**63**:9-17

[35] Verhoeckx KCM, Vissers YM, Baumert JL, Faludi R, Feys M, Flanagan S, et al. Food processing and allergenicity. Food and Chemical Toxicology : An International Journal published for the British Industrial Biological Research Association [Internet]. 2015;**80**:223-240. Available from: http://www.ncbi.nlm.nih.gov/pubmed/25778347 [Accessed: 1 April 2016]

[36] SAIFI, Maryam, SWAMY, Nithya, CRAIN, Maria, et al. Tolerance of a high-protein baked-egg product in egg-allergic children. Annals of Allergy, Asthma & Immunology, 2016;**116**(5):415-419

[37] Allen KJ, Remington BC, Baumert JL, Crevel RWR, Houben GF, Brooke-Taylor S, et al. Allergen reference doses for precautionary labeling (VITAL 2.0): Clinical implications. The Journal of Allergy and Clinical Immunology [Internet]. 2014;**133**(1):156-164. Available from: http://www.sciencedirect.com/science/article/pii/S0091674913010592 [Accessed: 26 April 2016]

[38] Muraro A, Hoffmann-Sommergruber K, Holzhauser T, Poulsen LK, Gowland MH, Akdis CA, et al. EAACI food allergy and anaphylaxis guidelines. Protecting consumers with food allergies: Understanding food consumption, meeting regulations and identifying unmet needs. Allergy [Internet]. 2014;**69**(11):1464-1472. Available from: http://doi.wiley.com/10.1111/all.12453 [Accessed: 15 March 2017]

[39] Downs ML, Taylor SL. Effects of thermal processing on the enzyme-linked immunosorbent assay (ELISA) detection of milk residues in a model food matrix. Journal of Agricultural and Food Chemistry [Internet]. 2010;**58**(18):10085-10091. Available from: http://pubs.acs.org/doi/abs/10.1021/jf101718f [Accessed: 22 November 2016]

[40] Sanchiz Á, Ballesteros I, Martin A, Rueda J, Pedrosa MM, Dieguez M del C, et al. Detection of pistachio allergen coding sequences in food products: A comparison of two real time PCR approaches. Food Control [Internet]. 2017;**75**:262-270. Available from: http://linkinghub.elsevier.com/retrieve/pii/S0956713516306880 [Accessed: 23 March 2017]

[41] Khuda S, Slate A, Pereira M, Al-Taher F, Jackson L, Diaz-Amigo C, et al. Effect of processing on recovery and variability associated with immunochemical analytical methods for multiple allergens in a single matrix: Sugar cookies. Journal of Agricultural and Food Chemistry [Internet]. 2012;**60**(17):4195-4203. Available from: http://www.ncbi.nlm.nih.gov/pubmed/22486175 [Accessed: 26 April 2016]

[42] Gomaa A, Boye JI. Impact of thermal processing time and cookie size on the detection of casein, egg, gluten and soy allergens in food. FRIN. 2013;**52**:483-489

[43] Iqbal A, Shah F, Hamayun M, Ahmad A, Hussain A, Waqas M, et al. Allergens of Arachis hypogaea and the effect of processing on their detection by ELISA. Food & Nutrition Research [Internet]. 2016;**60**:28945. Available from: http://www.pubmedcentral.nih.gov/articlerender.fcgi?artid=4773821&tool=pmcentrez&rendertype=abstract [Accessed: 26 April 2016]

[44] Benedé S, López-Expósito I, Molina E, López-Fandiño R, Boyce JA, Assa'ad A, et al. Egg proteins as allergens and the effects of the food matrix and processing. Food & Function [Internet]. 2015;**6**(3):694-713. Available from: http://xlink.rsc.org/?DOI=C4FO01104J [Accessed: 10 June 2016]

[45] Nesvizhskii AI. Protein Identification by Tandem Mass Spectrometry and Sequence Database Searching. In: Mass Spectrometry Data Analysis in Proteomics [Internet]. New Jersey: Humana Press; 2007. pp. 87-120. Available from: http://www.ncbi.nlm.nih.gov/pubmed/17185772 [Accessed: 24 March 2017]

[46] Sealey-Voyksner J, Zweigenbaum J, Voyksner R. Discovery of highly conserved unique peanut and tree nut peptides by LC–MS/MS for multi-allergen detection. Food Chemistry [Internet]. 2016;**194**:201-211. Available from: http://www.ncbi.nlm.nih.gov/pubmed/26471545 [Accessed: 8 March 2017]

[47] Shefcheck KJ, Musser SM. Confirmation of the allergenic peanut protein, Ara h 1, in a model food matrix using liquid chromatography/tandem mass spectrometry (LC/MS/MS). Journal of Agricultural and Food Chemistry [Internet]. 2004;**52**(10):2785-2790. Available from: http://www.ncbi.nlm.nih.gov/pubmed/15137814 [Accessed: 8 March 2017]

[48] Cucu T, De Meulenaer B, Devreese B. MALDI based identification of soybean protein markers – Possible analytical targets for allergen detection in processed foods. Peptides [Internet]. 2012;**33**(2):187-196. Available from: http://linkinghub.elsevier.com/retrieve/pii/S0196978111005183 [Accessed: 8 March 2017]

[49] MacLean B, Tomazela DM, Shulman N, Chambers M, Finney GL, Frewen B, et al. Skyline: An open source document editor for creating and analyzing targeted proteomics experi-

ments. Bioinformatics [Internet]. 2010;**26**(7):966-968. Available from: http://www.ncbi.nlm.nih.gov/pubmed/20147306 [Accessed: 15 March 2017]

[50] Mead JA, Bianco L, Ottone V, Barton C, Kay RG, Lilley KS, et al. MRMaid, the web-based tool for designing multiple reaction monitoring (MRM) transitions. Molecular & Cellular Proteomics [Internet]. 2009;**8**(4):696-705. Available from: http://www.ncbi.nlm.nih.gov/pubmed/19011259 [Accessed: 15 March 2017]

[51] Rogniaux H, Pavlovic M, Lupi R, Lollier V, Joint M, Mameri H, et al. Allergen relative abundance in several wheat varieties as revealed via a targeted quantitative approach using MS. Proteomics [Internet]. 2015;**15**(10):1736-1745. Available from: http://doi.wiley.com/10.1002/pmic.201400416 [Accessed: 20 December 2016]

[52] Hoofnagle AN, Whiteaker JR, Carr SA, Kuhn E, Liu T, Massoni SA, et al. Recommendations for the generation, quantification, storage, and handling of peptides used for mass spectrometry-based assays. Clinical Chemistry [Internet]. 2015;**62**(1):48-69. Available from: http://www.ncbi.nlm.nih.gov/pubmed/26719571 [Accessed: 10 March 2017]

[53] Heick J, Fischer M, Kerbach S, Tamm U, Popping B. Application of a liquid chromatography tandem mass spectrometry method for the simultaneous detection of seven allergenic foods in flour and bread and comparison of the method with commercially available ELISA test kits. Journal of AOAC International [Internet]. 2011;**94**(4):1060-1068. Available from: http://europepmc.org/abstract/med/21919338 [Accessed: 28 April 2016]

[54] Wang H, Tu Z-C, Liu G-X, Liu C-M, Huang X-Q, Xiao H. Comparison of glycation in conventionally and microwave-heated ovalbumin by high resolution mass spectrometry. Food chemistry [Internet]. 2013;**141**(2):985-991. Available from: http://www.ncbi.nlm.nih.gov/pubmed/23790877 [Accessed: 26 April 2016]

[55] Heick J, Fischer M, Pöpping B. First screening method for the simultaneous detection of seven allergens by liquid chromatography mass spectrometry. Journal of Chromatography A [Internet]. 2011;**1218**(7):938-943. Available from: http://www.ncbi.nlm.nih.gov/pubmed/21227428 [Accessed: 28 April 2016]

[56] PILOLLI, Rosa, DE ANGELIS, Elisabetta, et MONACI, Linda. Streamlining the analytical workflow for multiplex MS/MS allergen detection in processed foods. Food Chemistry, 2017;**221**:1747-1753

[57] Lamberti C, Cristina L, Acquadro E, Elena A, Corpillo D, Davide C, et al. Validation of a mass spectrometry-based method for milk traces detection in baked food. Food chemistry [Internet]. 2016;**199**:119-127. Available from: http://linkinghub.elsevier.com/retrieve/pii/S0308814615302776 [Accessed: 20 December 2016]

[58] Pedreschi R, Nørgaard J, Maquet A. Current challenges in detecting food allergens by shotgun and targeted proteomic approaches: A case study on traces of peanut allergens in baked cookies. Nutrients [Internet]. 2012;**4**(12):132-150. Available from: http://www.ncbi.nlm.nih.gov/pubmed/22413066 [Accessed: 10 March 2017]

[59] Huschek G, Bönick J, Löwenstein Y, Sievers S, Rawel H. Quantification of allergenic plant traces in baked products by targeted proteomics using isotope marked peptides. LWT - Food Science and Technology [Internet]. 2016;**74**:286-293. Available from: http://linkinghub.elsevier.com/retrieve/pii/S0023643816304674 [Accessed: 3 April 2017]

[60] Planque M, Arnould T, Dieu M, Delahaut P, Renard P, Gillard N. Advances in ultra-high performance liquid chromatography coupled to tandem mass spectrometry for sensitive detection of several food allergens in complex and processed foodstuffs. Journal of Chromatography A. 2016;**1464**:115-123

[61] Parker CH, Khuda SE, Pereira M, Ross MM, Fu T-J, Fan X, et al. Multi-allergen quantitation and the Impact of thermal treatment in industry-processed baked goods by ELISA and liquid chromatography-tandem mass spectrometry. Journal of Agricultural and Food Chemistry [Internet]. 2015;**63**(49):10669-10680. Available from: http://www.ncbi.nlm.nih.gov/pubmed/26595064 [Accessed: 23 September 2016]

[62] Gomaa A, Boye J. Simultaneous detection of multi-allergens in an incurred food matrix using ELISA, multiplex flow cytometry and liquid chromatography mass spectrometry (LC-MS). Food Chemistry [Internet]. 2015;**175**:585-592. Available from: http://www.ncbi.nlm.nih.gov/pubmed/25577123 [Accessed: 28 April 2016]

[63] Sayers RL, Johnson PE, Marsh JT, Barran P, Brown H, Mills ENC. The effect of thermal processing on the behaviour of peanut allergen peptide targets used in multiple reaction monitoring mass spectrometry experiments. The Analyst [Internet]. 2016;**141**(13):4130-4141. Available from: http://www.ncbi.nlm.nih.gov/pubmed/27113917 [Accessed: 8 March 2017]

[64] Campbell L, Raikos V, Euston SR. Modification of functional properties of egg-white proteins. Nahrung/Food [Internet]. 2003;**47**(6):369-376. Available from: http://doi.wiley.com/10.1002/food.200390084 [Accessed: 10 June 2016]

[65] Davis PJ, Williams SC. Protein modification by thermal processing. Allergy [Internet]. 1998;**53**(46 Suppl):102-105. Available from: http://www.ncbi.nlm.nih.gov/pubmed/9826012 [Accessed: 8 March 2017]

[66] Mueller GA, Maleki SJ, Johnson K, Hurlburt BK, Cheng H, Ruan S, et al. Identification of Maillard reaction products on peanut allergens that influence binding to the receptor for advanced glycation end products. Allergy [Internet]. 2013;**68**(12):1546-1554. Available from: http://www.ncbi.nlm.nih.gov/pubmed/24266677 [Accessed: 8 March 2017]

[67] Monaci L, Pilolli R, De Angelis E, Godula M, Visconti A. Multi-allergen detection in food by micro high-performance liquid chromatography coupled to a dual cell linear ion trap mass spectrometry. Journal of Chromatography A [Internet]. 2014;**1358**:136-144. Available from: http://www.ncbi.nlm.nih.gov/pubmed/25042441 [Accessed: 26 April 2016]

[68] Bignardi C, Mattarozzi M, Penna A, Sidoli S, Elviri L, Careri M, et al. A rapid size-exclusion solid-phase extraction step for enhanced sensitivity in multi-allergen determination in dark chocolate and biscuits by liquid chromatography–tandem mass spectrometry.

Food Analytical Methods [Internet]. New York: Springer. 2013;**6**(4):1144-1152. Available from: http://link.springer.com/10.1007/s12161-012-9521-4 [Accessed: 10 March 2017]

[69] Dumont V, Kerbach S, Poms R, Johnson P, Mills C, Popping B, et al. Development of milk and egg incurred reference materials for the validation of food allergen detection methods. Quality Assurance and Safety of Crops & Foods [Internet]. 2010;**2**(4):208-215. Available from: http://doi.wiley.com/10.1111/j.1757-837X.2010.00081.x [Accessed: 23 September 2016]

[70] Kirsch S, Fourdrilis S, Dobson R, Scippo M-L, Maghuin-Rogister G, De Pauw E. Quantitative methods for food allergens: A review. Analytical and Bioanalytical Chemistry [Internet]. 2009;**395**(1):57-67. Available from: http://link.springer.com/10.1007/s00216-009-2869-7 [Accessed: 20 December 2016]

[71] Lutter P, Parisod V, Weymuth H. Development and validation of a method for the quantification of milk proteins in food products based on liquid chromatography with mass spectrometric detection. Journal of AOAC International [Internet]. 2010;**94**(4):1043-1059. Available from: http://www.ncbi.nlm.nih.gov/pubmed/21919337 [Accessed: 20 December 2016]

[72] Bantscheff M, Schirle M, Sweetman G, Rick J, Kuster B. Quantitative mass spectrometry in proteomics: A critical review. Analytical and Bioanalytical Chemistry [Internet]. 2007;**389**(4):1017-31. Available from: http://www.ncbi.nlm.nih.gov/pubmed/17668192 [Accessed: 10 March 2017]

[73] Ong S-E, Mann M. Mass spectrometry–based proteomics turns quantitative. Nature Chemical Biology [Internet]. 2005;**1**(5):252-262. Available from: http://www.ncbi.nlm.nih.gov/pubmed/16408053 [Accessed: 10 March 2017]

[74] Paez V, Barrett WB, Deng X, Diaz-Amigo C, Fiedler K, Fuerer C, et al. AOAC SMPR(®) 2016.002. Journal of AOAC International [Internet]. 2016;**99**(4):1122-1124. Available from: http://www.ncbi.nlm.nih.gov/pubmed/27455945 [Accessed: 22 November 2016]

[75] Monaci L, van Hengel AJ. Development of a method for the quantification of whey allergen traces in mixed-fruit juices based on liquid chromatography with mass spectrometric detection. Journal of Chromatography A [Internet]. 2008;**1192**(1):113-120. Available from: http://www.ncbi.nlm.nih.gov/pubmed/18394633 [Accessed: 10 March 2017]

[76] Careri M, Costa A, Elviri L, Lagos J-B, Mangia A, Terenghi M, et al. Use of specific peptide biomarkers for quantitative confirmation of hidden allergenic peanut proteins Ara h 2 and Ara h 3/4 for food control by liquid chromatography–tandem mass spectrometry. Analytical and Bioanalytical Chemistry [Internet]. 2007;**389**(6):1901-1907. Available from: http://link.springer.com/10.1007/s00216-007-1595-2 [Accessed: 20 December 2016]

[77] Mattarozzi M, Bignardi C, Elviri L, Careri M. Rapid shotgun proteomic liquid chromatography–electrospray ionization–tandem mass spectrometry-based method for the lupin (*Lupinus albus* L.) multi-allergen determination in foods. Journal of Agricultural

and Food Chemistry [Internet]. 2012;**60**(23):5841-5846. Available from: http://www.ncbi.nlm.nih.gov/pubmed/22612429 [Accessed: 10 March 2017]

[78] Zhang J, Lai S, Zhang Y, Huang B, Li D, Ren Y. Multiple reaction monitoring-based determination of bovine α-lactalbumin in infant formulas and whey protein concentrates by ultra-high performance liquid chromatography-tandem mass spectrometry using tryptic signature peptides and synthetic peptide stand. Analytica Chimica Acta [Internet]. 2012;**727**:47-53. Available from: http://dx.doi.org/10.1016/j.aca.2012.03.034

[79] Posada-Ayala M, Alvarez-Llamas G, Maroto AS, Maes X, Muñoz-Garcia E, Villalba M, et al. Novel liquid chromatography–mass spectrometry method for sensitive determination of the mustard allergen Sin a 1 in food. Food Chemistry [Internet]. 2015;**183**:58-63. Available from: http://linkinghub.elsevier.com/retrieve/pii/S0308814615003428 [Accessed: 23 March 2017]

[80] Ahsan N, Rao RSP, Gruppuso PA, Ramratnam B, Salomon AR. Targeted proteomics: Current status and future perspectives for quantification of food allergens. Journal of Proteomics [Internet]. 2016;**143**:15-23. Available from: http://www.ncbi.nlm.nih.gov/pubmed/27113134 [Accessed: 10 March 2017]

[81] Brun V, Masselon C, Garin J, Dupuis A. Isotope dilution strategies for absolute quantitative proteomics. Journal of Proteomics [Internet]. 2009;**72**(5):740-749. Available from: http://linkinghub.elsevier.com/retrieve/pii/S1874391909001079 [Accessed: 23 March 2017]

[82] Newsome GA, Scholl PF. Quantification of allergenic bovine milk α_{S1}-casein in baked goods using an intact ^{15}N-Labeled protein internal standard. Journal of Agricultural and Food Chemistry [Internet]. 2013;**61**(24):5659-5668. Available from: http://www.ncbi.nlm.nih.gov/pubmed/22670623 [Accessed: 10 March 2017]

[83] Chen Q, Zhang J, Ke X, Lai S, Tao B, Yang J, et al. Quantification of bovine β-casein allergen in baked foodstuffs based on ultra-performance liquid chromatography with tandem mass spectrometry. Food Additives & Contaminants Part A, Chemistry, Analysis, Control, Exposure & Risk Assessment [Internet]. 2015;**32**(1):25-34. Available from: http://www.ncbi.nlm.nih.gov/pubmed/25413212 [Accessed: 09 March 2017]

[84] Liao Y-S, Kuo J-H, Chen B-L, Tsuei H-W, Lin C-Y, Lin H-Y, et al. Development and validation of the detection method for wheat and barley glutens using mass spectrometry in processed foods. Food Analytical Methods [Internet]. Springer US. 2017;1-9. Available from: http://link.springer.com/10.1007/s12161-017-0827-0 [Accessed: 23 March 2017]

[85] Planque M, Arnould T, Renard P, Delahaut P, Dieu M, Gillard N. Highlight on bottlenecks in food allergen analysis: Detection and quantification by mass spectrometry. Journal of AOAC International [Internet]. 2017; Available from: http://www.ingentaconnect.com/content/10.5740/jaoacint.17-0005 [Accessed: 15 March 2017]

[86] Chen J, Wang M, Turko IV. Quantification of amyloid precursor protein isoforms using quantification concatamer internal standard. Analytical Chemistry [Internet]. 2013;**85**(1):303-307. Available from: http://pubs.acs.org/doi/abs/10.1021/ac3033239 [Accessed: 05 April 2017]

[87] Chen Q, Zhang J, Ke X, Lai S, Li D, Yang J, et al. Simultaneous quantification of α-lactalbumin and β-casein in human milk using ultra-performance liquid chromatography with tandem mass spectrometry based on their signature peptides and winged isotope internal standards. Biochimica et Biophysica Acta (BBA): Proteins and Proteomics [Internet]. 2016;**1864**(9):1122-1127. Available from: http://linkinghub.elsevier.com/retrieve/pii/S1570963916301157 [Accessed: 10 March 2017]

[88] Korte R, Brockmeyer J. MRM3-based LC-MS multi-method for the detection and quantification of nut allergens. Analytical and Bioanalytical Chemistry [Internet]. 2016;**408**(27):7845-7855. Available from: http://link.springer.com/10.1007/s00216-016-9888-y [Accessed: 20 December 2016]

[89] Ippoushi K, Sasanuma M, Oike H, Kobori M, Maeda-Yamamoto M. Absolute quantification of Pru av 2 in sweet cherry fruit by liquid chromatography/tandem mass spectrometry with the use of a stable isotope-labelled peptide. Food Chemistry [Internet]. 2016;**204**:129-134. Available from: http://www.ncbi.nlm.nih.gov/pubmed/26988485 [Accessed: 28 March 2017]

[90] Abdel Rahman AM, Kamath SD, Gagné S, Lopata AL, Helleur R. Comprehensive proteomics approach in characterizing and quantifying allergenic proteins from northern shrimp: Toward better occupational asthma prevention. Journal of Proteome Research [Internet]. American Chemical Society. 2013;**12**(2):647-656. Available from: http://pubs.acs.org/doi/abs/10.1021/pr300755p [Accessed: 28 March 2017]

Chapter 3

Vegetable Proteins: Non-sensitizing Encapsulation Agents for Bioactive Compounds

Julián Quintero, Ana Naranajo, Gelmy Ciro and
John Rojas

Additional information is available at the end of the chapter

http://dx.doi.org/10.5772/intechopen.70378

Abstract

Plant-derived proteins are remarkable macromolecules of scientific interest because they represent an alternative to the animal-derived proteins and petroleum-derived polymers. Many food proteins especially those derived from animal sources could act as antigens in humans. For instance, milk proteins extracted from cows may cause food intolerance during infancy. Further, soybean, peanuts, tree nuts, fish, crustacean shellfish and egg proteins may act as antigens in 90% of children. Since the GI tract is permeable to intact antigens the oral intake of these proteins may generate gastrointestinal (50–80%), cutaneous (20-40%) and respiratory symptoms (4–25%). Most of these allergens are water-soluble glycoproteins that are resistant to acids and enzymes. Usually, these proteins have a small molecular weight (10,000–60,000 kDa), water solubility, glycosylation residues, and a relative resistance to heat and digestion. Allergenicity is less frequent in vegetable proteins due to their less flexible and non-compact structure. Allergenicity is also related to the resistance to proteolysis, post-translational glycosylation, presence of epitopes, and enzymatic proteolysis. Moreover, proteins serve as a coating material if structural modifications in the protein, either by physical, chemical or enzymatic mechanisms are conducted. As a result, their allergenicity is reduced, and their functional properties are enhanced.

Keywords: encapsulation agents, allergenicity, proteins, bioactive compounds, protein derivatization

1. Introduction

A food allergy occurs once the body develops a specific and repetitive immune response to certain foods [1]. It can be divided into two major categories based on the mechanism involved: (i) the immunoglobulin E (IgE)-mediated, such as allergy to proteins from milk, egg, peanut etc. It is the most severe reaction, especially to food containing proteins, and (ii) the non-IgE-mediated allergy such as that of gluten or celiac disease, where the allergic symptom is triggered by ingestion of gluten from cereals namely wheat, rye and barley in their diets. In recent years, food allergies have caused a major health alarm affecting nearly 1% of adult population in the world and from 6 to 8% of children [2–4]. Thus, the prevalence of food allergies has increased in several regions all over the world. Further, more than 170 types of foods have been identified as potentially allergenic [5]. The animal-derived sources include eggs, milk, fish and crustacean shellfish; whereas the vegetable-derived sources include wheat, soy and nuts. The former group of proteins are responsible for causing more than 90% of allergic reactions [5, 6]. Most food allergens are stable molecules that resist the effect of food processing, cooking and the digestive process. These glycoproteins are characterized by their ability to induce a pathogenic IgE response in susceptible individuals [7]. Usually, food allergens are formed by divalent or multivalent molecules with two or more antibodies–binding sites calls epitopes, which are responsible for interacting with immune effector molecules such as the IgE antibodies [2–4]. Moreover, many food proteins especially those derived from animal sources could act as antigens in humans.

Currently, there is a worldwide search for new materials of natural origin that confers the physical, chemical and sensory characteristics to food products similar to those of synthetic additives applied on a daily basis. These synthetic compounds have been considered as potentially toxic in hypersensitive people, leading to health problems, causing allergies, hyperactivity, and cancer [8–11].

Proteins are macromolecules considered as emergents, these are versatile compounds having a good biocompatibility, biodegradability, high nutritional value, amphiphilic properties, and exhibit a strong interaction with several types of active compounds via hydrogen bonds, and electrostatic interactions [12]. Further, proteins are also able to function as emulsifiers, foaming and gelling agents [13–16]. Their chemical and structural versatility makes them suitable candidates for the delivery of bioactive hydrophobic and hydrophilic ingredients from a wide range of platforms such as particles, fibers, films and hydrogels [16].

One of the emerging and promising uses of proteins is in the microencapsulation tecnology of different compounds in the pharmaceutical, food and cosmetic fields. This technology is defined as a mechanical, chemical or physico-chemical process that isolates and protects the potentially sensitive active ingredients (i.e., liquid, solid or gas) from the damaging environment. In most cases, spherically-shaped products are obtained and the resulting particles could be classified according to their size as capsules (1–1000 μm), microcapsules (100–1000 nm) or nanocapsules (1–100 nm). In this process, the active ingredient is protected from the environment by a membrane, which in turn is named as the wall or coating material. This membrane controls the release and stability of the core material [17]. Nonetheless, to date, only a few proteins have been considered to be effective coating materials for the encapsulation of several core compounds such as vitamins, minerals, microorganisms, oils, phenolic compounds, among others. These proteins are mainly obtained from animal sources rather than plant sources. Proteins derived from milk, wheat, soy and cereals are the most widely studied for this aplication, but are considered as allergenic. For this reason, research has focused on the search for new sources of nonallergenic proteins that allows for the modification of their physical structures using chemical treatments such as the Maillard, hydrolysis, acylation or cationization reactions to improve the encapsulating capacity of the protein and in turn, decrease their allergenicity.

2. Allergenic proteins

Proteins are macromolecules derived from plants or animals that range in size from several thousand to several million Daltons [18, 19]. In general, proteins are composed of amino acids linked through peptide bonds resulting in chain lengths ranging from ~50 to >100,000 amino acids [19]. This sequence creates a characteristic three-dimensional organization (or folding) which in turn, can be organized into four structural levels.

The primary structure of proteins is formed by the linear sequence of bound amino acids. The secondary structure is due to the formation of hydrogen bonds between the carbonyl (-CO-) and amino (-NH) groups forming a folded structure. The latter describes the path that the polypeptide backbone of the protein follows in the three dimentions. The alpha and beta helices are the most important conformations of the secondary structure. Further, the tertiary structure describes the three-dimensional organization of all atoms in the polypeptide chain, including the side groups, as well as the polypeptide backbone. The quaternary structure of the protein is formed by the association between two or more proteins that exhibit a tertiary structure, resulting in a typical functionality [19, 20].

Amino acids are amphoteric in nature and thus, react with acids or bases due to the presence of alkaline (NH_2) and acidic (COOH) groups. Currently, there are twenty common amino acids having side chains of different size, shape, charge and chemical reactivity [19, 20]. The degree of hydrophobicity and hydrophilicity of amino acids is one of the main determinants of the three-dimensional structure of proteins. Amino acids such as glycine, alanine, valine, leucine, isoleucine, methionine and proline have non-polar aliphatic side chains; whereas phenylalanine and tryptophan have non-polar aromatic side groups. These hydrophobic amino acids are generally found within proteins, forming the so called hydrophobic core [19]. Other amino acids have ionizable side chains such as arginine, aspartic acid, glutamic acid, cysteine, histidine, lysine, and tyrosine; whereas asparagine, glutamine, serine, and threonine contain non-ionic polar groups, which are often found on the surface of the protein allowing for a strong interaction with the aqueous ambient [19].

Proteins are mainly obtained from: (i) oilseeds and protein crops such as soybeans, rapeseed, peas, lentils, broad beans and sunflowers; (ii) cereal sources such as wheat, oats, rye, barley, maize, rice, sorghum, millet and quinoa; and (iii) algae [21]. Vegetable proteins also possess several advantages such as a good biodegradability and biocompatibility, have a low cost and a high availability, and pose no health risks [22, 23].

Proteins can be classified according to their sedimentation coefficient (S), which is defined as the rate of sedimentation per unit of acceleration of the particle in a medium. This property varies according to the molecular weight, conformational space and behavior of the protein in the environment. However, there are four large families of plant proteins that are classified according to their solubility into globulins, albumins, prolamins and glutelins. Albumin and globulins are the main constituents of plant-derived proteins [19].

Albumins are highly soluble in water and have a molecular weight ranging from 10 to 100 kDa. This group includes mostly proteins that present structural and storage functions [24]. In general, albumins contain high levels of lysine and sulfur amino acids, such as methionine and cysteine, and a high amount of disulfide bridges that favor the resistance against thermal denaturation [19, 20].

On the other hand, globulins are the main proteins obtained from vegetable sources. They are soluble in aqueous saline solutions and are mainly composed of two fractions having a sedimentation coefficient of 7S and 11S, respectively, which in turn depend on the plant source and culture conditions. Globulins are an important part of storage proteins, and have a molecular weight of more than 100 kDa. They are rich in arginine, aspartic acid, glutamic acid and their amides [19, 20].

Glutelins and prolamins are proteins soluble in basic aqueous solutions and hydroalcoholic mixtures, respectively. Their structure has been poorly studied, but these fractions represent agglomerates of globulins bound together by disulfide bonds and hydrophobic interactions, resulting in a complex morphology [21].

Currently, there are 16,712 recognized protein families in the Pfam database, but only 255 (~1.13%) of them are considered as allergens. Further, only 0.16% of the top 20 families account for ~80% of all reported cases of food allergenicity (**Table 1**) [25].

Further, it has been observed that the structural properties of proteins significantly affect their functionality, including the allergenic potential [25]. A survey conducted on common protein allergens reveals that they possess a wide range of physical characteristics, and none of them is unique to a class of protein allergens. Nevertheless, one report suggested that allergens tend to be ovoid in shape, although it is unclear why this should contribute

Family	Source	Family	Source
Prolamin superfamily	Plant	Oleosins	Plant
Tropomyosin	Animal	Lipocalin	Animal: arthropod and mammalian
Cupin superfamily	Plant	Beta-1,3-glucanase	Plant
Profilin	Plant	Papain-like cysteine protease	Plant
EF-hand domain	Plant, animal	Thaumatin-like protein	Plant
PR-10	Plant	Expansin, C-term	Plant: all grasses
Alpha/beta-caseins	Mammal	Trypsin-like serine proteases	Animal: arthropod and mammalian
Hevein-like domain	Plant	Enolase	Fungi and plants
Class I chitinases	Plant	Expansin, N-term	Plant: all grasses except 1

Table 1. Classification of allergenic proteins according to their family and source.

to allergenicity [26]. Further, the fact of having repetitive motifs also contribute to allergenicity [26]. Many of the important allergens are exceptionally heat stable and retain their allergenicity after heating [26]. However, there are proteins not considered as allergens that possess any of the properties described previously [26].

Particular claims have been made regarding the contribution of intramolecular disulfide bonds to the allergenicity of proteins. Thus, proteins from house dust mites could induce allergenicity if disulfide bonding through site-directed mutagenesis occurs. Otherwise, allergenicity prevents making proteins unable to bind IgE. Further, the loss of disulfide bonds may cause allergens to lose their immunologic identities (i.e., the ability to bind pre-existing specific IgE antibody) and hence, the ability to initiate the novo IgE production [26]. Further, the induction of IgE antibody by wheat agglutinin could be lessened by reducing disulfide bonds with thioredoxin [26]. However, the ability of disulfide bonds to have a qualitative contribution to the allergenicity of wheat agglutinin is still unknown. A quantitative reduction of the antigenicity of a protein could result in a reduction of the allergic response to a protein without altering its intrinsic allergenicity, only if the vigor of the immune response is reduced. In order to determine whether the intrinsic allergenicity of a protein has been altered, it is necessary to assess independently its allergenicity and its antigenicity. This may be achieved experimentally by simultaneously measuring both the IgE (allergenic) and IgG (antigenic) response upon exposure. Further, it seems likely that disulfide bonds influence allergenicity, in unpredictable ways. Their presence can profoundly affect the processing and stability of antigens, and hence the release or destruction of T-cell epitopes [26]. The presence of multiple intramolecular disulfide bonds *per se* does not make a protein as an allergen, nor does their absence preclude allergenicity. For instance, ovalbumin is considered as an allergen despite of having only a single intramolecular disulfide bond that contributes little to its stability, whereas bovine serum albumin (BSA) having 17 intramolecular disulfide bonds is much less allergenic [26].

2.1. Allergenic animal proteins

Animal food allergens are classified into three general families such as tropomyosins, EF-hand proteins, and caseins [27]. However, regardless of their family the ability to act as an allergen appears to be related to relative identity with human homologues. Thus, if the protein has a sequence identity from 54 to 63% with respect to human homologues, then it is considered as allergenic. Nevertheless, a higher identity does not implies allergenicity [27, 28].

The family of tropomyosins is divided into four types of muscle proteins, where none of them causes an IgE response in humans [25]. In fact, no human IgE response to tropomyosin from birds or fish has been identified. This is expected since these sequences have an identity with human tropomyosins greater than 63%, which is translated in the absence of allergenic activity [27].

EF proteins form the second family of animal-derived food allergens, and they are composed of parvalbumin [27]. Parvalbumins are divided into α- and β-parvalbumin. The α-parvalbumin is considered to be non-allergenic, whereas β-parvalbumin is found in a variety of fish species, retaining the allergenic potential and is absent in human muscle [28].

Out of the caseins that have been shown to elicit an IgE response in humans, the rule of thumb is the closer the sequence to the human equivalent is, the less likely an IgE response will occur. Conversely, sensitization to BSA is the main predictive marker for the cross-reactivity to cow's milk that is present in 73–93% of patients with beef allergies, despite of the fact that BSA shares 76% identity to its human homolog [27, 29].

Cow's milk and egg allergies are some of the most common food allergies found in young children. It is estimated that ~3.8 and 2% of children younger than 5 years old have cow's milk and egg allergies, respectively. These allergens are commonly found in a variety of foods due to their technological and nutritional importance [6]. Thus, lactoglobulin is the major allergen in cow´s milk. Milk contains more than 20 protein fractions. In the curd, four caseins account for ~80% of milk proteins. The remaining 20% of the proteins, are globular proteins (e.g., lactalbumin, lactoglobulin, and bovine serum albumin), and are found in whey and egg proteins from both components (i.e., yolk and egg white) causing sensitization [30].

Parvalbumin represents the major clinical cross-reactive fish allergen. It contains heat-resistant linear epitopes that are s sensitizing by the interaction of metal-binding domains. In addition, other fish allergens are found in collagen and gelatin isolated from skin and muscle tissues. On the other hand, in shellfish, crustaceans and mollusks, tropomyosin is the major allergen that triggers allergic reactions [31].

2.2. Allergenic vegetable proteins

About 65% of plant food allergens belong to the group of prolamins, termites and the group of proteins related to pathogenesis (PR-10) [25]. The prolamin family include storage proteins, lipid transfer (LTPs), alpha-amylase/protein inhibitors and albumins from most cereal seeds. Their 3D structure consists of a compact structure with four alpha-helices stabilized by disulfide bridges and a central cavity used for lipid binding. However, similarity in their third-party structures does not indicate a similarity in their amino acid sequence between proteins in the same group. Further, prolamins from wheat are known to cause baker's asthma and celiac disease in humans. Alpha-amylase/trypsin inhibitors from various cereals, such as wheat, barley and rice, have also been involved in allergies. Some of the clinically reported allergenic plant proteins belongs to the family of prolamins such as Ara h 2, Ara h 6, Sin a 1, Ber e 1, Ses i 2 and Jug v 1. Non-specific LTPs are known to be the main food allergens in the fruits of the *Rosaceae* family. The presence of specific IgE in LTP is considered a significant risk factor for allergy and may serve as a diagnostic marker [25]. The most relevant termite-type allergens are the 7S and 11S globulins. 7S globulins include Arah1, Jugr2 and Sesi3, whereas the 11S globulins include the Arah3, soy glycinins, Bere2, Cora9 and Fage1 [32]. The third structure of the proteins belonging to the termite group consists of a series of antiparallel β leaves associated with an α-helix forming a cavity [32]. This structure is also found in several lipocalin-like proteins involved in the transport of hydrophobic ligands, including milk β-lactoglobulin [32]. Further, plant prophylines share about 70% of the amino acid sequence homology [32–34].

All gliadin and glutenin protein fractions have been described as wheat grain allergens. The main properties of these proteins is to form a continuous viscoelastic network when flour is mixed with water to form a dough to be used in products such as bread, pastries, pasta, and crackers. However, wheat gluten exhibits a low solubility in aqueous solution. This fact limits the applications of wheat gluten in various types of food, since a good solubility is the main requirement for use in liquid foods and beverages. Furthermore, solubility is closely related to other functional properties of proteins such as the foaming, emulsifying, and gelling ability [35]. In soybean there are eight registered proteins which could trigger an allergic response. However, two of them named as β-conglycinin and glycinin represent ~70% of the soybean proteins. As a result, the incidence of soy protein allergy is much lower than other food allergens, such as milk or peanut proteins [36].

There are over 10 allergenic proteins identified in peanuts of which the Ara h 1, Ara h 2, and Ara h 3 are the most abundant peanut allergens and cumulatively represent approximately half of the total protein content [37]. Furthermore, the prevalence of allergy to tree nuts is estimated to be about half of that of peanut allergy. Tree nut allergic reactions tend to be severe and accidental exposures are common. Walnut, cashew, almond, pecan, Brazil nut, hazelnut, macadamia nut, pistachio, and pine nut are the most common tree nuts responsible for allergy cases in the USA and Europe. Moreover, from 20 to 50% of peanut allergic patients are also allergic to tree nuts [38].

3. Mechanism of action of allergenic proteins

The prevalence of food allergy has been steadily increasing around the world. The relevant risk factors for food allergies are: (i) an increased use of antacids which is translated in a reduced digestion of allergens; (ii) a reduced consumption of omega-3 polyunsaturated fatty acids in the diet; (iii) a reduced consumption of antioxidants; (iv) genetics; (v) male gender; (vi) race, since it is increased among asian and black children as compared to white children; (vii) an increased hygiene; (viii) a northern climate; (ix) obesity, since this is an inflammatory state; (x) timing and route of exposure to foods (increased risk for delaying allergens with possible environmental sensitization); and (xi) vitamin D insufficiency [1, 39]. Most food allergens belong to only a limited number of proteins, and around 65% of plant food allergens belong to just four protein families, such as the prolamin, cupin, Bet v 1-like, and profiling, whilst animal food allergens can be classified into three main families named as tropomyosins, EF-hand proteins and caseins [40]. In general, children food allergies to milk, egg, wheat, and soy typically resolve during childhood, whereas allergies to peanut, tree nuts, fish, and shellfish are persistent. The prognosis also varies with disorder; for instance, food allergy related to eosinophilic esophagitis appears to have a relatively poor chance of resolution. For instance, the resolution rates are slow for allergies that have been commonly outgrown, such as those to milk, egg, wheat, and soy [39].

The human body has a series of physiological barriers for protection against foreign antigens. In the digestive system, these barriers are composed of two groups: (i) non-immunological such as the gastric acid, pancreatic enzymes, intestinal enzymes, mucus, the membrane of the microvilli, the mucosal layer and intestinal peristalsis), and (ii) immunological, such as IgA, IgE, IgM, IgG, lymphocytes, macrophages, Peyer's patches, intestinal secretory IgA and secretory IgA in breast milk [30]. Usually, when the immune system recognizes food proteins as a foreign body, immunoregulatory mechanisms are established that lead to the acquisition of tolerance. Alterations in these regulatory mechanisms alter the induction of tolerance, resulting in food allergy [30]. An allergy reaction require a complex interaction between the protein and the immune system [26]. The National Institute of Allergy and Infectious Diseases of the United States, identified four categories of immune-mediated adverse food reactions such as IgE-mediated, non–IgE-mediated, mixed, and cell-mediated reactions. The most prevalent non-IgE-mediated reactions are eosinophilic esophagitis (EoE), the food-protein induced enterocolitis syndrome, proctocolitis, entheropathy and celiac disease [41]. The IgE-mediated reaction is by far, the most well established mechanism, where the antibodies bind to the high affinity receptors of mast cells and basophils, and to the low affinity receptors on macrophages, monocytes, lymphocytes and platelets. Thus, IgE are able to bind a specific receptor on the surface of mast cells and basophils, when two or more of these captive IgE molecules bind to their specific antigen, becoming cross-linked on the surface of the cell [26]. Once the allergens penetrate the mucosal barriers and bind to the IgE of mast cells and basophils, these cells release mediators that cause vasodilatation, smooth muscle contraction and mucosal secretion, giving rise to the typical symptoms of immediate hypersensitivity (**Annex 1**) [30].

In order to crosslinking to takes place, at least two antibody molecules must bind to the inducing allergen. An allergen must therefore contain at least two IgE binding sites, each one contains at least 15 amino acid residues. This implies a lower size limit for protein allergens of approximately 30 amino acid residues [26]. The IgE-mediated allergic immune response can be divided into three phases: (i) the sensitization phase in which B lymphocytes switch to the production of specific IgE, (ii) the effector phase consisting of an acute reaction and a facultative late-phase reaction; (iii) a chronic phase that may be the result of repetitive late phase reactions. The acute reaction causes activation of mast cells and basophils releasing histamine, leukotrienes, and other mediators known to be responsible for the wheal and flare reaction occurring in the skin and at various mucosal sites including the eye, nose, lung, and gastrointestinal tract [7]. The IgE-mediated reaction occur immediately or within 1–2 h of ingestion, whereas non-IgE–mediated reactions generally have a delayed onset beyond 2 h of ingestion [42].

A limited number of foods are responsible for the majority of reactions in IgE-mediated food allergy. For instance, allergy to cow milk, eggs, wheat, and soy are more common

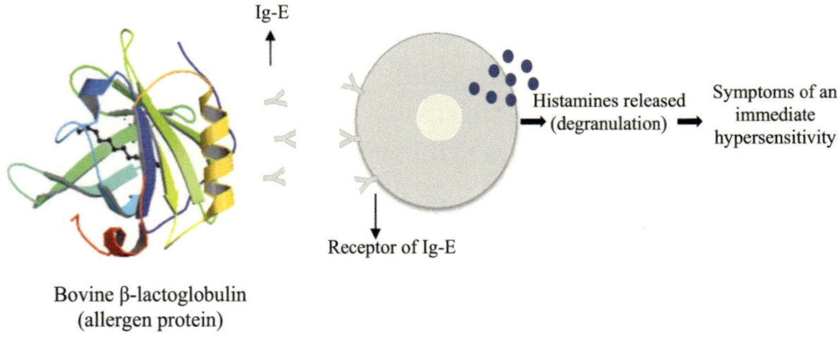

Annex 1. IgE-mediated protein hypersensitivity.

in infants and young children, whereas seafood, peanuts, and tree nuts are the most common causes of food allergy in adults [40]. The IgE-mediated reaction in skin includes hives and angioedema, whereas the gastrointestinal manifestations include mouth and lip pruritus, abdominal pain, vomiting, and diarrhea. On the other hand, a variety of respiratory tract symptoms that generally involve IgE-mediated responses, includes rhinorrhea and wheezing, whereas isolated asthma or rhinitis are unusual [42]. Further, the IgE-mediated food allergy may cause the dietary protein–induced syndromes such as enteropathy and enterocolitis. These in turn, cause profuse vomiting, diarrhea, dehydration and lethargy. Other syndromes include proctocolitis, gastroesophageal reflux, infantile colic, constipation and the Heiner syndrome [42].

4. Proteins used as coating materials: an emergent trend

There are many coating materials considered as "generally regarded as safe (GRAS)" which are used in the encapsulation process. Most of them are derived from natural sources such as natural gels (e.g., gum arabic, alginates, carrageenan and mesquite gum), modified starches, maltodextrin and proteins (e.g., whey proteins, gelatin, soy, rice, sunflower and peas) [13, 18, 43–49].

Animal-derived proteins are the most widely used coating materials, either alone or in complexes with polysaccharides applying techniques such as coacervation and spray drying. For instance, Chi and City [50] used whey protein to encapsulate rambutan oil by spray drying. They obtained an EE and yield of 69.9 and 28.5%, respectively using gelatin as a coating material; whereas whey proteins rendered an EE of 73.9% and yield of 58.6%. The best yield and EE was achieved with milk proteins instead of proteins obtained from tissues. Likewise, several researchers have evaluated the encapsulation activity of proteins such as gelatin [19, 45, 51], sodium caseinate in combination with lactose, or maltodextrin and other protein-carbohydrate complexes [19]. Remarkably, Rubio and his team [52] patented the process to obtain microcapsules and nanocapsules based on free whey proteins or complex polysaccharides employing "Blow-spinning," "blow-spraying," "electrospinning" and "electrospraying" as encapsulation techniques. In general, animal proteins tend to be more soluble, flexible and smaller in size at a broader pH range than proteins obtained from plant sources. For instance, casein proteins have a molecular mass of 20 kDa, whereas the molecular mass of soy proteins is 350 kDa. Further, animal proteins have a much faster diffusion kinetics at the interfaces and present a greater stability in emulsions, which is the key in many encapsulation processes [12, 53]. On the other hand, the large globular nature of vegetable proteins presents a greater challenge at stabilizing the interface in an emulsion and these proteins render a low EE. These emulsions are stabilized by increasing the viscosity of the continuous phase instead of acting on the interface, leading to a lower entrapment efficiency of the dispersing compound resulting in a higher susceptibility towards oxidative and degradation reactions. However, plant proteins exhibit several advantages that make them highly attractive in the pharmaceutical, cosmetic and food fields [12, 53]. For instance, plant proteins reflect the current "green" and "clean" label trends, and they are not considered allergenic as compared to the animal-derived proteins. In addition, the niche marketing restrict the use of animal proteins in the diet and increase their cost promoting plant proteins as ideal coating materials from more abundant sources [12, 53].

In order to replace synthetic polymers and animal-derived products, there is a growing interest in the industrial use of renewable resources from natural origin having unexplored applications. Thus, natural macromolecules such as plant proteins have drawn considerable attention due to their availability, biodegradability, renewable character and various physicochemical properties that make them able to form films. The film forming ability of proteins is based on the unfolding characteristics of the protein structure in a solvent. This unfolding is favored by pH changes, addition of electrolytes, heat treatments, or solvent removal [13, 19, 20, 43, 54–56]. The solvents used to prepare the protein solutions are mostly water, ethanol, and rarely acetone. Proteins must be in an open or extended form in order to allow the molecular interactions for the formation of the film to take place. Further, these interactions depend on the protein structure (degree of extension) and the respective sequence of hydrophobic and hydrophilic amino acids in the protein. Therefore, vegetable proteins are very suitable materials for the encapsulation process of active ingredients in the food, pharmaceutical and cosmetic fields [12, 46, 53].

4.1. Encapsulation methods with proteins

Since the encapsulation methods are diverse and complex, they are classified according to the type of organic solvent, the energy expenditure, or application field. However, the most common classification method is related to the production process. In this case, it could be classified as physical, chemical or physicochemical processes [46, 57]. In general, the encapsulation process involves three steps: (i) the formation of a wall around the core material; (ii) complete closure of the wall, so any possible leakage of the core is avoided; (iii) generation of a capsule, either by chemical reactions or physical treatments [58]. The particle shape thus obtained depends on the physicochemical properties of the core, the coating material and the technique implemented (**Figure 1**) [21].

The morphology (shape and structure) of the microparticles is in turn, classified into two categories: capsules and spheres [18]. In the first case, the capsule is composed of a cluster of particles having a liquid or solid core surrounded by a continuous solid coating, which is generated only by chemical methods. In the second type, the sphere is formed mechanically, either by a process of atomization or milling process. Whereby, the active ingredients are finely dispersed as fine solid particles or liquid droplets within the matrix. A third category may rise comprising more complex structures, such as multilayer capsules or multilayer spheres. Further, both capsule and spherical morphologies should not have defects or pinholes to ensure a greater stability. Therefore, the presence of defects may increase the rate of oxidation or hydrolytic degradation (**Figure 1**) [18, 53]. Further, microparticles might exhibit from irregular to spherical shape. In fact, the coating material is generally adapted to the outline of the particle having a wide variety of shapes [21].

The most common encapsulation techniques include spray drying, extrusion, coacervation, liposome formation, fluid bed coating, inclusion complexes, ionic gelation, lyophilization, cocrystallization and emulsification. As mentioned previously, their morphology is classified into two major categories named as microspheres and microcapsules. Microspheres are typically

http://dx.doi.org/10.5772/intechopen.70378

Encapsulation technique	Morphology obtained
Spray-drying	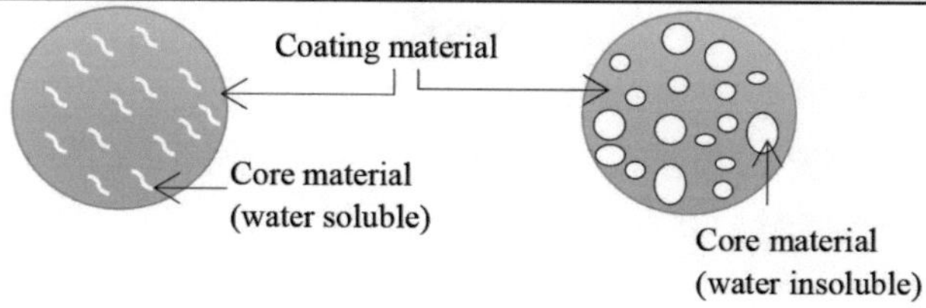
Coacervation	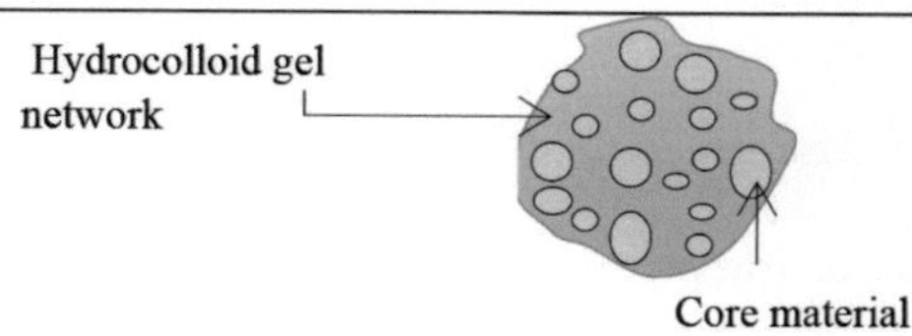
Emulsion (o/w or w/o)	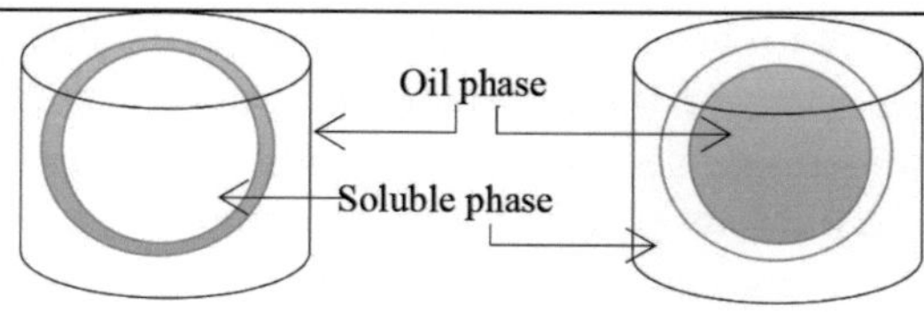

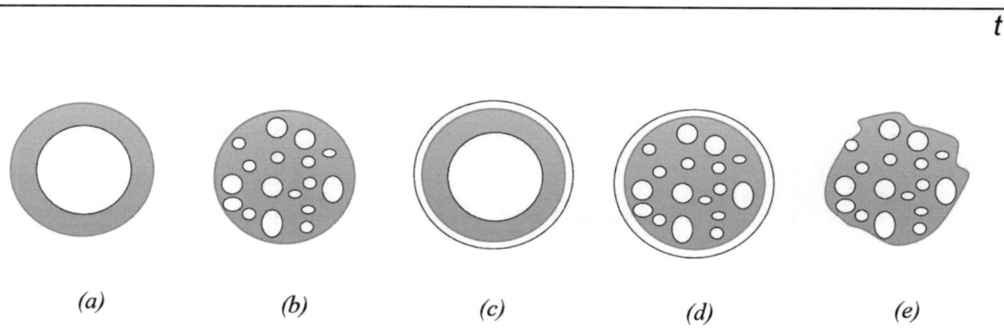

Figure 1. Morphology of the particles obtained by microencapsulation: (a) single microcapsule, (b) microsphere, (c) multilayer microcapsule, (d) multilayer microspheres, and (e) irregular microcapsule.

formed by a physical process such as spray drying, fluid bed coating, extrusion, and multiple emulsification [18, 59, 60]. On the other hand, the chemical process associated to the capsule formation include phase separation, ionic gelation, coacervation and liposome formation [18, 44, 57]. The different methods used for microencapsulation and the resulting main features are presented in **Table 2**.

The choice of the encapsulation technique for a particular process depends on: (i) the desirable size, biocompatibility and biodegradability of the particles; (ii) the physicochemical properties of the core and the coating materials; (iii) the intended use; (iv) the desired release mechanism from the core; and (v) the production costs. Some of the most commonly used encapsulation techniques which employ proteins as the coating material are described as follows:

Encapsulation method	Particle size (μm)	Max. load (%)	Type of process	Reference
Simple coacervation	20–200	<60	Chemical	[61]
Complex coacervation	5–200	70–90	Chemical	[61]
Co-current spray drying	1–100	<40	Physical	[21]
Counter-current spray drying	50–200	10–20	Physical	[21]

Table 2. Properties of the microcapsules produced by different techniques.

4.1.1. Emulsification

The emulsification process involves the formation of colloidal systems formed by two immiscible liquids in which the dispersed phase is in the form of small droplets (i.e., between 0.1 and 10 μm) distributed in a continuous or dispersing phase. Emulsions are unstable if they are allowed to stand for some time. As a result, the molecules of the dispersed phase are redistributed forming a layer that can precipitate or migrate to the surface depending on the density gradient between the two phases [21]. In general, emulsions are classified according to the continuous phase when one liquid is dispersed into another. For instance, an O/W emulsion is formed when a hydrophobic liquid is dispersed in water or in a water-soluble liquid. On the contrary, a W/O emulsion is formed when a water-soluble liquid is dispersed in a hydrophobic solvent [57]. Moreover, the stabilization process of the emulsions is achieved by three mechanisms:

i. Formation of a strong emulsifier layer or film around the individual droplets of the suspended liquid;

ii. Formation of an electrostatically charged layer on the surface of the individual droplets;

iii. Viscosity increase of the dispersant medium. Thus, as the viscosity of the dispersant liquid increases, the Brownian motion slows down decreasing the probability of particles to agglomerate. As a result, the sedimentation rate of the particles or their possible flocculation rate is reduced.

One of the mostly widely used strategies to achieve the stabilization of emulsions is by the incorporation of surfactants in the system. These compounds have amphiphilic (i.e., hydrophilic and hydrophobic) regions in their structure and hence, they have the ability to reduce the interfacial tension between the phases of the emulsion system leading to a better stability [62]. Polysaccharides are the most commonly used emulsifiers and are mainly represented by native and denatured starches, phospholipids and proteins. Plant protein properties such as water solubility, amphiphilicity, the ability to self-associate and interact with a variety of substances, a high molecular weight and flexibility make them ideal for encapsulation by emulsification followed by techniques such as spray drying, coacervation, ionic gelation and solvent evaporation [21].

The absorption and emulsifying properties of the proteins at the interface of the colloidal system depend on many factors such as protein structure, state of aggregation, pH, and ionic strength [63]. For instance, caseins, which have a random spiral conformation, tend to form an interweaved layer; whereas whey proteins that are globular in shape usually form aggregates at the interface of the colloidal system [64]. Further, bovine serum albumin, whey protein and proteins isolated from plant sources such as soybean, pumpkin seed, quinoa and peas have been used as emulsifiers in many encapsulation systems, including W/O and W1/O/W2 double emulsions [65–67]. Proteins could also be combined with other emulsifiers to stabilize emulsions. In fact, protein-polysaccharide complexes having electrostatic interactions between molecules of opposite charge at a certain pH and ionic strength range could stabilize emulsions. For instance, the sodium caseinate/soybean lecithin complex is an stable emulsion which is used to encapsulate phenolic compounds, simultaneously [68].

4.1.2. Spray drying

Microencapsulation by spray drying is the most widely known technique used to encapsulate food ingredients such as vitamins (C and E), fragrances, probiotic bacteria, lipids, vegetable oils, minerals (i.e., iron), anthocyanin pigments, milk, and foodstuffs [45, 47, 48, 60, 69]. The technique of microencapsulation by spray drying has been used since the 1950s and is currently applied at the industrial and academic level due to its rapid speed, economy and simplicity. It involves the dispersion of the active ingredient with the encapsulation material that is pumped into a spray chamber followed by dehydration with circulating hot air at a temperature between 150 and 200°C [45, 47, 48, 60, 69]. Spray drying provides a relatively high EE as compared to other methods. The highest EE achieved with spray drying is between 96.0 and 100.0%, which is much higher than those obtained with alternative methods [18]. Several parameters need to be controlled during the spray drying process. The inlet and outlet drying air temperatures, the feed flow of the product, the residence time and the characteristics of the raw material are the most important factors [18]. The initial mixture needs to be in a form of a dispersion, a solution, or an O/W emulsion having a low viscosity. The process is divided into different stages:

i. Atomization of the feed mixture;

ii. Interaction of the liquid phase with hot air;

iii. Evaporation of the droplets;

iv. Separation of the formed microcapsules.

The ideal materials for spray drying should have a low viscosity at high concentrations, a high solubility, have a good emulsifying and film forming ability, and hold efficient thermal properties (i.e., low effective diffusivity and low conductivity) to protect the encapsulated material during the drying process [21]. Thus, the drying process can be carried out following three different patterns: (i) co-current, if the solution is atomized in the same direction than the hot air flow (**Figure 2a**); (ii) countercurrent, if the sprayed microdroplets move in the opposite path than the flow of hot air (**Figure 2b**); and (iii) mixed, if the spray droplets move without a defined trajectory and at a high entropy. Thus, the air flow moves in opposite and/or concurrent directions (**Figure 2c**).

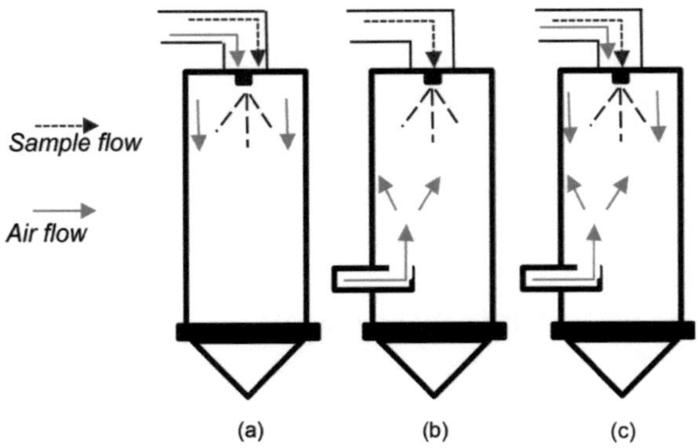

Figure 2. Spray-drying pattern types: (a) co-current, (b) counter-current, and (c) mixed.

The average particle size obtained by the atomization process varies between 1 and 100 μm for the co-current and between 50 and 200 μm for the counter-current drying pattern [21].

4.1.3. Coacervation

Coacervation is a chemical method of phase separation. The term "coacervation" was introduced in the colloid chemistry field by Bungenberg de Jong and Kruyt in 1929 to describe the spontaneous separation of the liquid/liquid phases that can occur when polyelectrolytes of opposing charges are mixed in an aqueous medium [17, 44, 70–73]. Coacervation is defined by the International Union of Pure and Applied Chemistry (IUPAC) as the separation of a colloidal system into two liquid phases. Thus, coacervation is an intermediate state between dissolution and precipitation and hence, it leads to a partial desolvation in opposition to the exhaustive solvation associated to the process of precipitation. Therefore, any factor that involves polymer desolvation causes the coacervation phenomenon [53]. The coacervation-triggering phenomena include temperature changes, pH modification and the addition of an incompatible anti-solvent, salt or another polymer [18, 53]. The coacervation procedure can be classified into two types: (i) simple or (ii) complex coacervation, depending on the number of polymers involved [18]. Complex coacervation mainly occurs by electrostatic interactions between two or more solutions of opposite-charged polymers producing two immiscible liquid phases: (i) one is the continuous phase having a low polymer concentration, whereas, the second one is composed of the polymer rich dense phase, also named as the coacervate phase, which in turn is used to coat a variety of active core ingredients. Usually, the coacervate complexes possess the combined functional properties of each polymer involved [21]. On the other hand, simple coacervation only implies one polymer, and thus, it is not very popular in the food and pharmaceutical fields [18, 43]. In general, the process of coacervation involves the following steps:

i. Dispersion: A vigorous stirring of the active ingredient (liquid or solid particles) is carried out in a solution of the polymer, or a mixture of polymers that will form the wall material;

ii. Induction: Coacervation is induced by one of the previously described phenomena. The system of the solution becomes transparent and under the microscope the coacervate droplets have an appearance similar to that of an emulsion;

iii. Deposition: The adsorption of the coacervate droplets around the core material takes place. The cloudy supernatant is clarified as the process of coacervation evolves;

iv. Coalescence: Microscopic droplets of the coacervate form a continuous layer around the core;

v. Hardening: The system is subjected to cooling and a crosslinking agent is added to render a stiff shell (optionally);

vi. Separation: Microcapsules are isolated by centrifugation or filtration. Thus, spherical microcapsules as small as 4 μm are obtained having a large loading capacity (i.e., 90.0%).

4.2. Structural changes in proteins: a strategy to enhance their functionality

In recent years, the demand for multifunctional products has increased, and researchers need to develop or modify techniques to improve the functionality of proteins since most of them show no variability in their desirable functional properties [12, 19, 21]. Even though proteins are versatile materials with interesting properties, it may be necessary to modify the inherent properties such as solubility, hydrophobicity, hydrophilicity, the gelling, emulsifying, foaming and allergenicity. As a result, a versatile material is obtained, with less allergenicity and a wide variety of applications in different fields [12, 19, 21]. Several modifications can be conducted in proteins since amino acids have side chains of different sizes, shapes, charges and chemical reactivity. The reactivity of a protein, in terms of its ability to be chemically modified will be largely determined by the composition and location of the amino acids on its three-dimensional structure. These modifications can be made by physical (i.e., pressure and temperature), chemical or enzymatic methods [19]. Some of the feasible modifications of proteins are illustrated in **Annex 2**.

The term "crosslinking" is commonly used to describe the intra or inter-covalent bonding of a protein. As a result, the molecular size and shape, and the functional properties may be affected by crosslinking. Crosslinking can also be used for the stabilization and subsequent modulation of the release properties of the protein-based controlled release systems. Different methods can be used for crosslinking purposes, ranging from physical to enzymatic and chemical modifications [46, 74]. Crosslinking can be controlled by the proper reaction mechanism, reactive groups of the protein, and type of crosslinking reagent. The number of reactive groups per protein chain, types of functional groups, and spacer length of the crosslinking agent determine the resulting crosslinking density. The most relevant physical modifications of proteins imply variations in temperature and pressure that lead to structural changes or their denaturation. The main disadvantage of the heat treatment as a crosslinking method is that the reaction is difficult to control. The denaturation process of proteins begins when the structure itself becomes an intermediate product. As the reaction progress, the structure is altered, but the secondary structure remains unchanged. Once the chains unfold completely, the denaturation process is concluded. The magnitude of these changes depends on the protein source and environmental conditions (e.g., pH, solvent, presence of salts, surfactants, etc.) [75]. The more reactive the reducing sugar is the stronger and darker the gel becomes [12, 43, 46, 56, 76].

The enzymatic modification of proteins is another useful method. Various enzymes have the ability to crosslink proteins. Examples thereof include transglutaminase (TG), disulphide

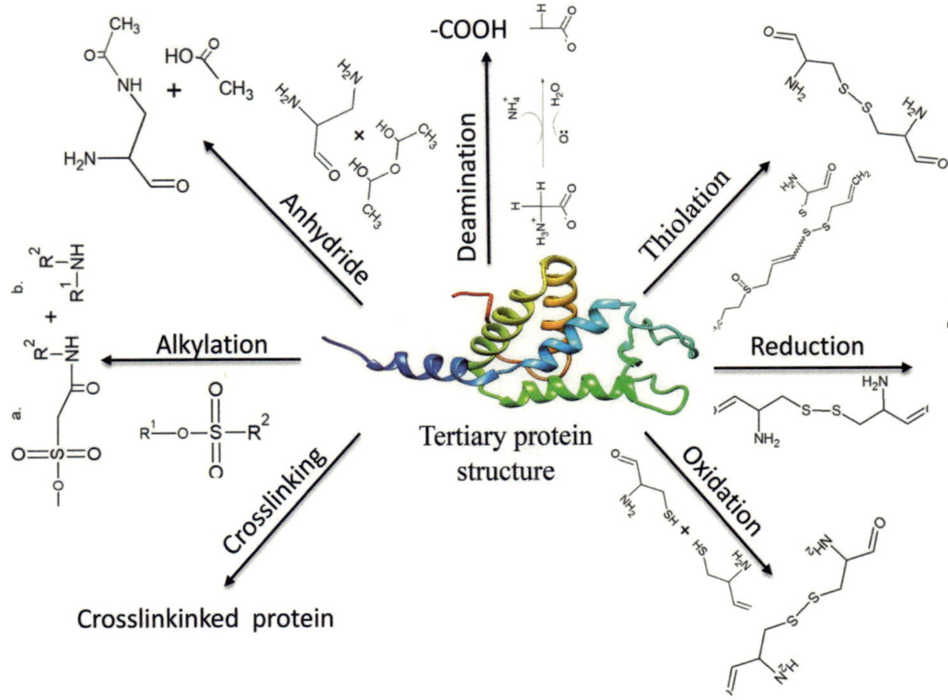

Annex 2. Schematic representation for the typical chemical modifications of proteins.

isomerase, peroxidase, lipoxygenase, and catechol oxidase. In a recent overview on enzymatic crosslinking, microbial TG, lactoperoxidase and glucose oxidase are highlighted as the enzymes available on a sufficient large scale for industrial applications [19]. TG is an acyltransferase that catalyzes the introduction of c-(y-glutamyl)-lysine crosslinks into proteins, making TG an interesting enzyme for food grade protein crosslinking. TG has been used to crosslink several proteins [19]. In general, caseins appear to be more susceptible to TG-induced crosslinking than whey-proteins, possibly due to the predominantly random structure of caseins, in contrast to the globular structure of whey proteins [19]. A less known type of crosslinking involves the peroxidase-catalyzed reaction between the side chains of two tyrosines, resulting in a C-C bond between the two carbons in an ortho position with respect to the phenol group [19]. This type of crosslinking is very strong due to the intermolecular formation of bonds. The use of co-substrates to enhance the crosslinking efficiency of peroxidases reduces the amount of enzyme needed and therefore increases the cost effectiveness. The co-substrates are phenolic compounds such as mono- and di-hydroxy benzene derivatives (e.g., catechol, ferulic acid, and *p*-hydroxybenzoic acid) and probably act as a spacer between the protein molecules [19].

On the other hand, the chemical modification of proteins has been the most widely studied method among scientists. These reactions are mainly represented by deamidation, acylation, chemical hydrolysis, and cationization reactions. There is a plethora of research conducted on the use of chemical agents for protein crosslinking [19]. The most widely used reagents are bifunctional having two reactive groups that can be used to introduce inter- and/or intramolecular bonds into proteins [19]. These reagents in turn, can be classified as homobifunctional or heterobifuntional. Homobifunctional reagents (i.e., glutaraldehyde) have two identical functional groups, whereas heterobifunctional reagents have two different functional groups. It is difficult to control the reaction conditions (i.e., pH, ionic strength and protein:reagent ratio) of homobifunctional reagents to ensure an intra- or intermolecular crosslinking. On the other hand, heterobifunctional reagents can be used in a more discriminating way. In this case, crosslinking occur in separate sequential steps, and the formation of intermolecular crosslinks can be avoided or stimulated. Tannins are complex polyphenolic substances that can be derived from galls, but also from fruits (e.g., pomegranate) and tea. Tannic acid (TA) is capable of complexing or crosslink proteins by forming a multiple hydrogen bonds network [19]. Proteins can hereby be physically crosslinked and thus, become more resistant to enzymatic degradation. This type of crosslinking is partially reversible. Further, some metal ions can oxidize TA and proteins, whereas other metals could inhibit the formation of hydrogen bonds.

All of these reactions modify the secondary or tertiary structure of the proteins using different compounds that could form linear biopolymers, biopolymers with hydrophobic linkage aggregates outside the structure, cationic or anionic biopolymers, or biopolymers in which certain specific amino acids are exposed. All of these modifications allow for an effective interaction of protein derivatives at the interface of emulsions, or with the active compound in the core, resulting in an improved EE. On the other hand, a protein could loss its original conformation or bonding which is responsible for its allergenicity, e.g., formation of disulfide bonds, which are responsible for binding the IgE and hence, triggering allergenicity.

Currently, many researchers are searching for alternatives to improve the encapsulation properties of vegetable proteins isolated from legumes (e.g., soybeans, peas, chickpeas and lentils), sunflower seeds and cereals (e.g., oats, wheat, barley and corn) [19–21, 44, 71, 77]. The chemical and enzymatic hydrolyses, the acylation [21], cationization [21, 78] and Maillard reactions [12, 19, 77] are the best chemical treatments to improve their functionality [12, 43]. For instance, Nesterenko et al. [46] studied native and modified soybean and sunflower seed proteins to encapsulate α-tocopherol by spray drying. Likewise, the EE increased from 82.6% for native soy protein to 94.8% for the modified product. Moreover, the EE of the native sunflower seed protein was 79.7%, whereas that of the acylated proteins was 99.5%. They concluded that the structural modification of the proteins increased the affinity between the active ingredient and the coating material, improving the encapsulation process, hydration and net protein load. Similar results were obtained by Chen Lia et al. 2015 [76], who encapsulated oleoresin obtained from tomato using soybean proteins conjugated with gum arabic as the coating material. These chemical modifications produced by Maillard reactions were conducted by heating at 60°C and at a relative humidity of 79% for 3, 6 and 9 days. They obtained EE of 69.25, 76.47, 80.91 and 84.69% for the native and modified proteins treated for 3, 6 and 9 days, respectively. The 3D change in the protein structure favors the stabilization of the emulsions, the encapsulation process and improves their biocompatibility.

Author details

Julián Quintero, Ana Naranajo, Gelmy Ciro and John Rojas*

*Address all correspondence to: jrojasca@gmail.com

College of Pharmaceutical and Food Sciences, University of Antioquia, Medellín, Colombia

References

[1] Grief SN. Food allergies. Primary Care: Clinics in Office Practice. 2016;**43**(3):375-391

[2] Jackson WF. Food Allergy. Concise monograph series. ILSI Press, International Life Sciences Institute. 2003.

[3] Prescott S, Pawankar R. A global survey of changing patterns of food allergy burden in children. World Allergy Organization Journal. 2013;**6**:21

[4] Ajala A, Cruz A, Faria J, Walter E, Granato D. Food allergens: Knowledge and practices of food handlers in restaurants. Food Control. 2010;**21**(10):1318-1321

[5] Houben G, et al. Prioritisation of allergenic foods with respect to public health relevance report from an ILSI Europe Food Allergy Task Force Expert Group. Food and Chemical Toxicology. 2016;**89**:8-18

[6] Manti S, et al. Breastfeeding and IL-10 levels in children affected by cow's milk protein allergy: A restrospective study. Immunobiology. 2017;**222**(2):358-362

[7] Bittencourt AL, et al. Immunogenicity and allergenicity of 2S, 7S and 11S soy protein fractions. Revista Brasileira de Ciências Farmacêuticas. 2007;**43**(4):597-606

[8] Demeyer D, Honikel K, De Smet S. The World Cancer Research Fund report 2007: A challenge for the meat processing industry. Meat science. 2008;**80**(4):953-959

[9] Viuda M, et al. In vitro antioxidant and antibacterial activities of extracts from annatto (*Bixa orellana* L.) leaves and seeds. Journal of Food Safety. 2012;**32**(4):399-406

[10] Mineo H, Ohdate T, Fukumura K. Effects of benzoic acid and its analogues on insulin and glucagon secretion in sheep. European Journal of Pharmaceutics and Biopharmaceutics. 1995;**280**(2):149-154

[11] Herrmann S, Duedahl-Olesen L, Granby K. Occurrence of volatile and non-volatile N-nitrosamines in processed meat products and the role of heat treatment. Food Control. 2015;**49**:163-169

[12] Zhang Y, et al. The effect of soy protein structural modification on emulsion properties and oxidative stability of fish oil microcapsules. Colloids and Surfaces B: Biointerfaces. 2014;**120**:63-70

[13] Avramenko NA, Chang C, Low NH, Nickerson MT. Encapsulation of flaxseed oil within native and modified lentil protein-based microcapsules. Food Research International. 2016;**81**:17-24

[14] Chang C, Varankovich N, Nickerson MT. Microencapsulation of canola oil by lentil protein isolate-based wall materials. Food Chemistry. 2016;**212**:264-273

[15] Li XR, Tang CH. Influence of glycation on microencapsulating properties of soy protein isolate-lactose blends. Journal of the Science of Food and Agriculture. 2013;**93**(11): 2715-2722

[16] Wan Z-L, Guo J, Yang X-Q. Plant protein-based delivery systems for bioactive ingredients in foods. Food & Function. 2015;**6**(9):2876-2889

[17] Jain A, Thakur D, Ghoshal G. Microencapsulation by complex coacervation using whey protein isolates and gum acacia: An approach to preserve the functionality and controlled release of β-carotene. Food and Bioprocess Technology. 2015;**8**(8):1635-1644

[18] Kasapis S, Norton IT, Ubbink JB. Modern Biopolymer Science: Bridging the Divide between Fundamental Treatise and Industrial Application. Academic Press. 2009

[19] Nedovic V, Willaert R. Fundamentals of Cell Immobilisation Biotechnology (Vol. 8). Springer Science & Business Media. 2013

[20] Gaonkar A G, Vasisht N, Khare A R, & Sobel R. Microencapsulation in the food industry: a practical implementation guide. Elseiver. 2014

[21] Nesterenko A, Alric I, Silvestre F, Durrieu V. Comparative study of encapsulation of vitamins with native and modified soy protein. Food Hydrocolloids. 2014;**38**:172-179

[22] Karaca AC, Nickerson M, Low NH. Microcapsule production employing chickpea or lentil protein isolates and maltodextrin: Physicochemical properties and oxidative protection of encapsulated flaxseed oil. Food Chemistry. 2013;**139**(1-4):448-457

[23] Pierucci APTR, Andrade LR, Baptista EB, Volpato NM, Rocha-Leão MHM. New microencapsulation system for ascorbic acid using pea protein concentrate as coat protector. Journal of Microencapsulation. 2006;**23**(6):654-662

[24] Qi PX, Onwulata CI. Physical properties, molecular structures, and protein quality of texturized whey protein isolate: Effect of extrusion temperature. Journal of Agricultural and Food Chemistry. 2011;**59**(9):4668-4675

[25] Masilamani M, Commins S, Shreffler W. Determinants of food allergy. Immunology and Allergy Clinics of North America. 2012;**32**(1):11-33

[26] Huby RDJ, Dearman RJ, Kimber I. Why are some proteins allergens?. Toxicological Sciences. 2000;**55**(2):235-246

[27] Jenkins J, Breiteneder H, Mills E. Evolutionary distance from human homologs reflects allergenicity of animal food proteins. Journal of Allergy and Clinical Immunology. 2007;**120**(6):1399-1405

[28] Wild L, Lehrer S. Fish and shellfish allergy. Current Allergy and Asthma Reports. 2005;**5**(1):74-79

[29] Restani P, Beretta B, Fiocchi A, Ballabio C, Galli CL. Cross-reactivity between mammalian proteins. Annals of Allergy, Asthma & Immunology. 2002;**89**(6):11-15

[30] Martorell A, Alonso E, Boné J, Echeverría L, López MC, Martín F, et al. Position document: IgE-mediated allergy to egg protein. Allergologia et Immunopathologia. 2013;**41**(5):320-336

[31] Abdel Rahman AM, Helleur RJ, Jeebhay MF, Lopata AL. Characterization of seafood proteins causing allergic diseases. Intech; 2012. pp. 107-140

[32] Marković-Housley Z, et al. Crystal structure of a hypoallergenic isoform of the major birch pollen allergen Bet v 1 and its likely biological function as a plant steroid carrier. Journal of Molecular Biology. 2003;**325**(1):123-133

[33] Hoffmann-Sommergruber K, Mills EC. Food allergen protein families and their structural characteristics and application in component-resolved diagnosis: New data from the EuroPrevall project. Analytical and Bioanalytical Chemistry. 2009;**395**(1):25-35

[34] Witke W. The role of profilin complexes in cell motility and other cellular processes. Trends in Cell Biology. 2004;**14**(8):461-469

[35] Battais F, Richard C, Jacquenet S, Denery-Papini S, & Moneret-Vautrin D A. Wheat grain allergies: an update on wheat allergens. European annals of allergy and clinical immunology. 2008;**40**(3):67

[36] Van Huis A, Dunkel FV. Soy protein: Impacts, production, and applications. In: Sustainable Protein Sources; 2016. pp. 23-45

[37] Nadathur S, Wanasundara J P D, & Scanlin L. Peanut products as a protein source: Production, nutrition, and environmental impact. In: Sustainable Protein Sources. 2016. pp. 209-221

[38] Skripak JM, Wood RA. Peanut and tree nut allergy in childhood. Pediatric Allergy and Immunology. Jun. 2008;**19**(4):368-373

[39] Sicherer SH, Sampson HA. Food allergy: Epidemiology, pathogenesis, diagnosis, and treatment. The Journal of Allergy and Clinical Immunology. 2014;**133**(2):291-307.e5

[40] Mills C. What makes an antigen a food allergen?. Clinical and Translational Allergy. 2011;**1**(Suppl 1):S2

[41] Lozano-Ojalvo D, Lezmi G, Cortes-Perez N, & Adel-Patient K. Non-IgE mediated food allergy. Drug Discovery Today: Disease Models. 2016;**17-18**:45-53

[42] Kattan JD, Cocco RR, Järvinen KM. Milk and soy allergy. Pediatric Clinics of North America. 2011;**58**:407-426

[43] Tamm F, Herbst S, Brodkorb A, Drusch S. Functional properties of pea protein hydrolysates in emulsions and spray-dried microcapsules. Food Hydrocolloids. 2016;**58**:204-214

[44] Jain A, Thakur D, Ghoshal G, Katare OP, Shivhare US. Characterization of microcapsulated β-carotene formed by complex coacervation using casein and gum tragacanth. International Journal of Biological Macromolecules. 2016;**87**:101-113

[45] Nakagawa K, & Fujii Y. Protein-based microencapsulation with freeze pretreatment: Spray-dried oil in water emulsion stabilized by the soy protein isolate-gum acacia complex. Drying Technology. 2015;**33**(13):37-41

[46] Nesterenko A, Alric I, Violleau F, Silvestre F, Durrieu V. The effect of vegetable protein modifications on the microencapsulation process. Food Hydrocolloids. 2014;**41**:95-102

[47] Bustamante M, Villarroel M, Rubilar M, Shene C. *Lactobacillus acidophilus* La-05 encapsulated by spray drying: Effect of mucilage and protein from flaxseed (*Linum usitatissimum* L.). LWT: Food Science and Technology. 2014;**62**:1162-1168

[48] Deng XX, Chen Z, Huang Q, Fu X, Tang CH. Spray-drying microencapsulation of alfa-carotene by soy protein isolate and/or OSA-modified starch. Journal of Applied Polymer Science. 2014;**131**(12):1-10

[49] Tang CH, Li XR. Microencapsulation properties of soy protein isolate: Influence of preheating and/or blending with lactose. Journal of Food Engineering. 2013;**117**(3):281-290

[50] Chi H, City M. Microencapsulation of rambutan seed oil by spray-drying using different protein preparations. International Food Research Journal. 2016;**23**(1):123-128

[51] Yúfera M, Fernández-Díaz C, Pascual E. Food microparticles for larval fish prepared by internal gelation. Aquaculture. 2005;**248**(1-4):253-262

[52] Rubio A, Cabello JM. Method for the production of micro-, sub-micro- and nano-capsules, based on milk serum proteins, WO2012/175776A1; 2013

[53] Can Karaca A, Low NH, Nickerson MT. Potential use of plant proteins in the microencapsulation of lipophilic materials in foods. Trends in Food Science & Technology. 2015;**42**(1):5-12

[54] Thakur MK, Thakur VK, Gupta RK, Pappu A. Synthesis and applications of biodegradable soy based graft copolymers: A review. ACS Sustainable Chemistry & Engineering. 2016;**4**(1):1-17

[55] Evans M, Ratcliffe I, Williams PA. Emulsion stabilisation using polysaccharide-protein complexes. Current Opinion in Colloid & Interface Science. 2013;**18**(4):272-282

[56] Liu F, Chen Z, Tang CH. Microencapsulation properties of protein isolates from three selected *Phaseolus* legumes in comparison with soy protein isolate. LWT: Food Science and Technology. 2014;**55**(1):74-82

[57] Zhang C, Li X, Liu Y-N, Zhang F. Utilization of microcapsule technology in foods. Journal of Nanoscience and Nanotechnology. 2015;**15**(12):9330-9340

[58] Fang Z, Bhandari B. Encapsulation of polyphenols—A review. Trends in Food Science & Technology. 2010;**21**(10):510-523

[59] Zhang Y, Tan C, Abbas S, Eric K, Xia S, Zhang X. Modified SPI improves the emulsion properties and oxidative stability of fish oil microcapsules. Food Hydrocolloids. 2015;**51**:108-117

[60] Kent RM, Doherty SB. Probiotic bacteria in infant formula and follow-up formula: Microencapsulation using milk and pea proteins to improve microbiological quality. Food Research International. 2014;**64**:567-576

[61] Madene A, Jacquot M, Scher J, Desobry S. Flavour encapsulation and controlled release—A review. International Journal of Food Science and Technology. 2006;**41**(1):1-21

[62] Wang S, et al. Application of nanotechnology in improving bioavailability and bioactivity of diet-derived phytochemicals. The Journal of Nutritional Biochemistry. 2014; **25**(4):363-376

[63] Livney YD. Milk proteins as vehicles for bioactives. Current Opinion in Colloid & Interface Science. 2010;**15**(1-2):73-83

[64] Augustin MA, Hemar Y. Nano- and micro-structured assemblies for encapsulation of food ingredients. Chemical Society Reviews. 2009;**38**(4):902-912

[65] Rayner M, MarkuD, Eriksson M, Sjöö M, Dejmek P, & Wahlgren M. Biomass-based particles for the formulation of Pickering type emulsions in food and topical applications. Colloids and Surfaces A: Physicochemical and Engineering Aspects. 2014;**458**(1):48-62

[66] Elsohaimy SA, Refaay TM, Zaytoun MAM. Physicochemical and functional properties of quinoa protein isolate. Annals of Agricultural Science. 2015;**60**(2):297-305

[67] Bucko S, Katona J, Popovis L, Vactag C, Petrovic L, Vucinice-Vasic M. Investigation on solubility, interfacial and emulsifying properties of pumpkin (*Cucurbita pepo*) seed protein isolate. LWT: Food Science and Technology. 2015;**64**(2):609-615

[68] Jia Z, Dumont MJ, Orsat V. Encapsulation of phenolic compounds present in plants using protein matrices. Food Bioscience. 2016;**15**:87-104

[69] Noshad M, Mohebbi M. Microencapsulation of vanillin by spray drying using soy protein isolate–maltodextrin as wall material. Flavour and Fragrance Journal. 2015;**30**:387-391

[70] Eratte D, McKnight S, Gengenbach TR, Dowling K, Barrow CJ, Adhikari BP. Co-encapsulation and characterisation of omega-3 fatty acids and probiotic bacteria in whey protein isolate-gum Arabic complex coacervates. Journal of Functional Foods. 2015;**19**:882-892

[71] Dong D, Qi Z, Hua Y, Chen Y. Microencapsulation of flaxseed oil by soya proteins–gum arabic complex coacervation. International Journal of Food Science and Technology. 2015;**50**:1785-1791

[72] Eratte D, Wang B, Dowling K, Barrow CJ, Adhikari BP. Complex coacervation with whey protein isolate and gum arabic for the microencapsulation of omega-3 rich tuna oil. Food & Function. 2014;**5**(11):2743-2750

[73] Xiao Z, Liu W, Zhu G, Zhou R, Niu Y. A review of the preparation and application of flavour and essential oils microcapsules based on complex coacervation technology. Journal of the Science of Food and Agriculture. 2014;**94**(8):1482-1494

[74] Jancurová M, Minarovičová L, Dandár A. Quinoa—A review. Czech Journal of Food Sciences. 2009;**27**(2):71-79

[75] Nesterenko A, Alric I, Silvestre F, Durrieu V. Vegetable proteins in microencapsulation: A review of recent interventions and their effectiveness. Industrial Crops and Products. 2013;**42**(1):469-479

[76] Lia C, Wang J, Shi J, Huang X, Peng Q, Xueb F. Encapsulation of tomato oleoresin using soy protein isolate-gum aracia conjugates as emulsifier and coating materials. Food Hydrocolloids. 2015;**45**:301-308

[77] Carbonaro M, Maselli P, Nucara A. Structural aspects of legume proteins and nutraceutical properties. Food Research International. 2014;**76**:19-30

[78] Teng Z, Xu R, Wang Q. Beta-lactoglobulin-based encapsulating systems as emerging bioavailability enhancers for nutraceuticals: A review. RSC Advances. 2015;**5**(44):35138-35154

Chapter 4

Antihistaminic Treatment, Allergen-Specific Immunotherapy, and Blockade of IgE as Alternative Allergy Treatments

Olga Lima Tavares Machado,
Débora Mothé de Campos-Mesquita and
Thais Pacheco-Soares

Additional information is available at the end of the chapter

http://dx.doi.org/10.5772/intechopen.69912

Abstract

Allergies mediated by immunoglobulin E (IgE) are the most common immunological hypersensitivity diseases. The prevalence has been continuously increasing in recent decades, and more than 25% of the population is currently affected. Symptoms of allergies can be observed in the skin and respiratory and gastrointestinal tracts, and systemic manifestations include anaphylactic shock. If an allergy is not properly diagnosed and treated, it tends to progress to a severe and chronic debilitating disease. Understanding the mechanisms by which the immune system induces and controls allergic inflammation depends on knowing the structure of several allergens and identifying epitopes, which are critical for the design of new strategies for treating allergies. Strategies for immunotherapy will be reviewed. Allergen-specific immunotherapy has been used for nearly a century and remains one of the few antigen-specific treatments for inflammatory diseases. There is a strong rationale for improving the efficacy of allergen-specific immunotherapy by reducing the incidence and severity of adverse reactions mediated by IgE. Approaches to address this problem, including the use of modified allergens, synthetic peptides as vaccines, and alternative strategies for blocking IgE, will be discussed.

Keywords: IgE blocker, antihistaminic, immunotherapy

1. Allergic mechanism

An allergen is defined as a normally harmless substance, found in the environment or food, which can produce asthma, fever, eczema, or gastrointestinal discomfort upon contact with a previously sensitized person. An allergy is commonly defined as an immediate or type I hypersensitivity reaction where symptoms appear rapidly and are caused by exposure to exogenous macromolecules known as antigens or allergens. The hypersensitivity reaction has two phases: sensitization, when the subject is first exposed to the antigen, and the subsequent reaction, when the subject is again exposed to the antigen [1]. **The first sensitization** of a body begins with the first contact with an antigen, which induces an allergy. The allergen penetrates the airways of the body or other tissues and is found by antigen-presenting cells (APCs) such as macrophages and/or dendritic cells, which encyst and proteolytically cleave the foreign substance. The peptide fragments generated, known as T cell epitopes, are directed to the outer membrane of the APC by the major histocompatibility class II (MHC II) complex in the form of a complex peptide-MHC class II [2]. The T-helper lymphocytes (Th1 and/or Th2) recognize these exposed epitopes and together with B cells initiate the immune response. The activation clones specific for the antigen, Th2 cells, are essential for the development of atopic diseases, because these cells activated by contact with APCs produce cytokines and interleukins 4 (IL-4) and 5 (IL-5). These interleukins act as signals, among other functions, for the biosynthesis of immunoglobulin E (IgE) by B lymphocytes. An immunoglobulin, IgE, binds to the surface of mast cells and basophils by FcЄRI receptors. A subsequent exposure to the same antigen, **the second sensitization**, leads to a substantial allergic response. The antigen-specific segments (IgE epitopes) are cross-linked to the IgE bound to the mast and/or basophil cells after interaction with the allergen, activating intracellular messengers, and the subsequent release of cellular mediators such as histamine and prostaglandins, which in turn induce physiological and anatomical changes that trigger the allergic symptoms of immediate hypersensitivity [3, 4].

IgE antibodies generated in response to a specific allergen interact with this allergen and trigger a series of intracellular reactions leading to the release of histamine and other inflammatory mediators. Histamine plays a key role in the allergic response. The release of histamine causes the smooth muscles of the gastrointestinal and respiratory tracts to contract, stimulates nerves, and dilates blood vessels [5, 6]. These effects of histamine include, among other clinical manifestations, erythema, flushing, nasal congestion, pruritus, headache, hypotension, tachycardia, and bronchoconstriction [5]. There are four main subtypes of histamine receptors: H1, H2, H3, and H4. These receptors are G-protein-coupled receptors that transfer extracellular signals via G proteins, acting as intermediates between cell-surface receptors and second intracellular messengers [6, 7]. The H1 receptor is the main mediator subtype of the allergic response causing allergic symptoms. In addition to its role in the immediate allergic response, histamine contributes to the late allergic response by stimulating the production of cell-adhesion molecules, class II antigens, and cytokines [6].

2. Tolerance induction

Immune tolerance can develop against any substance, and multiple mechanisms are involved. The lack of response of immune tolerance can lead to the development of various diseases such as:

- allergies
- asthma
- tumors
- chronic infections
- transplant organ rejection
- graft versus host disease
- many autoimmune diseases [8].

The generation of regulatory T (Treg) cells initiates tolerance. Peripheral tolerance is initiated by the secretion of IL-10 and TGF-β by allergen-specific Treg cells during continuous exposure. The induction of allergen-specific tolerance is associated with an increase in FOXP3+CD25+CD3+ cells in the nasal mucosa [9]. Atopic individuals have a reduced capacity to proliferate CD25+ and CD4 Treg cells, which indicates the mechanisms of failure of tolerance allergens. A clonal shift occurs during tolerance fromTh1, Th2 to Th1 (**Table 1**). B cells are stimulated by the action of IL-10 to produce IgG (particularly IgG4) and to suppress IgE production, which prevents the development of allergic symptoms in the tolerogenic individual [9–11] (**Table 2**).

If an allergy is not properly diagnosed and treated, it tends to progress to a severe and chronic debilitating disease.

Many treatments have been developed to circumvent the symptoms of allergic diseases, most of which use histamine inhibitors that mask the symptoms of the allergy. Allergen-specific immunotherapy (ASIT), however, is the only long-term preventive and long-term treatment for allergic diseases. ASIT involves the administration of a specific allergen, so it induces a specific immunological tolerance to the allergen. ASIT has been used for more than 100 years, but the mechanism of action has only recently been resolved [12].

IL-10	Inhibits the production of proinflammatory cytokines and the activation of Th2 and Th1
TGF-β	Inhibits the proliferation and differentiation of B and T lymphocytes
IgG4	Blocking antibody that inhibits the activation of effector cells by affecting the binding of allergen to IgE at Fcε receptors on the membranes of mast cells and basophils
HR2	Negatively regulates Th1- and Th2-type responses; these are G-protein-associated histamine receptors, which regulate various immunological events due to cAMP formation. Histamine induces the production of IL-10 by DC and Th2 and enhances the secretory activity of TGF in T cells

Table 1. Molecules with effector functions in allergen tolerance.

Treg	Secretors of TGF-β and IL-10; induce Foxp3 expression, Th2 suppression; direct, and indirect suppression of mast cells, basophils, and eosinophils; stimulate B lymphocytes in IgG4 production and IgE suppression
Breg	Expression of IL-10 and IgG4
Eosinophils Basophils Mast cells	Decrease the activity of inflammatory mediator secretion (histamine and leukotrienes) by the action of IL-10 and TGF secreted by regulatory cells

Table 2. Roles of cells in allergen tolerance.

In this chapter, we will describe the most common allergy treatments using antihistamines and emphasize the new methodologies of allergen-specific immunotherapy (ASIT) as a prophylactic treatment and IgE blockade as a therapeutic treatment.

3. Approaches for allergy treatment

3.1. Antihistaminic treatment

Researchers have devoted their efforts for many years to the development of effective and safe strategies for the treatment of allergy to alleviate the symptoms triggered by the body's responses to allergens [1, 13, 14]. Antihistamines are currently the most commonly used treatment. These drugs are used to alleviate allergic symptoms, that is, they are based on the consequences of the allergy [5]. First-generation antihistamines, or H1-receptor antagonists, may have undesirable side effects on the central nervous system, even at therapeutic doses, due to their ability to cross the blood-brain barrier rather than to their lack of selectivity. Side effects include sleepiness, sedation, and fatigue that may lead to reduced cognitive, memory, and psychomotor performance [7, 15]. First-generation antihistamines include doxepin, diphenhydramine, pyrilamine, chlorpheniramine, hydroxyzine, promethazine, and cyproheptadine [6].

A new class of antihistamine has been developed. Second-generation H1 antagonists cannot cross the blood-brain barrier as easily and have a greater affinity to H1 receptors, decreasing their sedative effects compared to the first-generation drugs [7]. These antihistaminic agents include cetirizine, ebastine, epinastine, fexofenadine, loratadine, desloratadine, levocetirizine, and rupatadine. The second-generation antihistamines cause fewer adverse effects, but some drugs, for example, levocetirizine, may cause drowsiness, and fexofenadine has a brief effect and may require more than one daily dose. Treatment with antihistaminic drugs does not address the cause of allergic responses but only alleviates their symptoms [7, 14, 16].

3.2. Allergen-specific immunotherapy (ASIT)

Immunotherapy was first conceived in 1911, from which a type of therapy was developed that used allergens as a tool for the development of immunological tolerance in sensitized individuals [17]. The term "desensitization" was replaced with "hypo-sensitization." The term "immunotherapy" became popular only in the 1980s and "specific immunotherapy" is a commonly used term. When immunotherapy involves the direct use of allergens as immunotherapeutics, the appropriate term is ASIT [12]. ASIT has been used for more than a century and remains one of the few antigen-specific treatments for inflammatory diseases.

ASIT consists of the gradual administration of doses of a specific allergen or part of that allergen to reduce the sensitivity and consequently to decrease the symptomatic reactions to a future exposure of the allergic individual to the causative natural agent [1, 18]. ASIT is a widely used therapeutic strategy for treating allergic rhinitis, venom-induced hypersensitivity, some drug allergies, and mild bronchial asthma [13]. The mechanisms of ASIT are not yet clear but include modulating both T and B cell responses, thereby reducing the incidence and severity of IgE-mediated adverse reactions [19]. Some of the immunological changes that occur during ASIT have been elucidated [1]. ASIT increases the level of allergen-specific IgA and IgG4 antibodies and decreases the level of allergen-specific IgE antibodies. Oral, sublingual, and subcutaneous immunotherapies are used the most in the treatment of hypo-sensitization in various types of allergies. These three mechanisms of immunotherapies, however, are specific to particular allergens, so the therapy is effective only for the particular allergen.

Approaches to improving ASIT include the use of modified recombinant allergens, novel adjuvants, and alternative routes of administration. Recombinant allergens are similar to wild-type allergens, generally equivalent in structure and properties, but with alterations in their epitopes that do not guarantee their ability to trigger an allergic response [20].

3.2.1. Recombinant hypoallergenic peptides for immunotherapy

Valenta et al. using purified recombinant allergens and derivatives of recombinant hypoallergenic allergens has identified the induction of the production of IgG-specific allergen-blocking antibodies as one of the main mechanisms of ASIT [21]. Blocking IgG, however, may also inhibit the presentation of antigen in APCs to antigen T cells and therefore suppress the activation of T cells induced [22]. ASIT can also alter the balance of specific helper T cells from a Th2 profile to an allergen-specific Th1 immunity profile and can induce the secretion of immunoregulatory cytokines such as interleukin (IL)-10, and regulatory T cells [23]. The induction of allergen-specific tolerance is thus the essential immune mechanism of ASIT.

Recombinant hypoallergenic from variants have been produced. Linhart constructed, purified, and characterized two hybrid hypoallergenic recombinant proteins from *Brassica rapa* allergens, Der p 2 (rder p 2)/1 C and rder p 2/1S [19]. Mutations in aspartic acid residues in these allergens decreased the cross-linking of IgE in the membrane of sensitized mast cells by decreasing the allergenic potential of the protein [24].

Patients immunized in 2016 with a variant Bet v1 (birch allergen) hypoallergen did not develop a local allergic response, as observed by histopathological tests of skin contact. Rats immunized with the same recombinant hypoallergen demonstrated that a profile of tolerogenic responses with proinflammatory cytokine production was possible [25].

3.2.2. Synthetic peptides

Immunotherapy using peptides has some advantages over immunotherapies fusing recombinant allergens. Vaccines using peptides with T cell epitopes can induce regulatory T cells.

The use of synthetic peptides derived from allergens containing T cell epitopes is an alternative to the production of allergen-specific T cells in ASIT. These peptides are formed from linear sequences representing fragments of small allergens that bind to the allergen-specific T cell receptor and do not react with IgE antibodies, which give them an advantage because they do not trigger the classic allergic symptoms measured by IgE. The treatment may induce T cell tolerance by the secretion of the immune cytokine regulator IL-10 from regulatory T cells. The diversity of T cell epitopes is a possible disadvantage of vaccines based on T cell epitopes, making treatment with only one or a few peptides difficult. This treatment can cause secondary systemic symptoms and lacks the ability to induce IgG blocking [2].

Vaccines for allergies based on B cell epitopes of approximately 20–40 amino acids use peptides that lack the ability to bind IgE. The peptides must be covalently linked to a protein transporter that is unrelated to the T allergens in order to render these peptides immunogenic, capable of inducing the production of IgG, which blocks the binding of IgE to the corresponding allergen. Valenta et al. demonstrated the use of carrier-linked allergenic peptides to induce IgG antibodies to the main pollen allergen of thyme grasses, Phl p 1, and to the main birch pollen allergen, Bet v 1. These conjugates decreased allergenic activity even more than the recombinant hypoallergens, because the non-IgE-reactive peptides were selected from the IgE-binding sites [21].

3.3. Allergen-nonspecific therapy

3.3.1. Anti-IgE antibodies

The new approaches for the treatment of allergic diseases have two main strategies using nonspecific allergens [26]. The first strategy is to bind IgE to high-affinity receptors (FcεRI) in mast cells and basophils, and the second strategy is to interfere with the signaling generated by receptor binding (FcεRI) [26, 27]. Knowledge of the pathophysiological role of IgE antibodies has allowed the development of new drugs against many allergic diseases.

3.3.2. Anti-IgE receptor antibodies

A currently promising therapeutic approach has been the use of antibodies against the region of the IgE molecule that interacts with specific IgE receptors. The interaction of IgE molecules with high- and low-affinity receptors may be inhibited by the use of anti-IgE for reducing the induced allergic responses, preventing the activation of mast cells and consequently the release of allergic mediators [2, 26]. Omalizumab is a murine anti-human IgE monoclonal antibody that binds to the same receptor site (Cε3) to which IgE binds, thereby inhibiting the binding of IgE-to-IgE receptors [2, 8]. Omalizumab does not bind to fixed IgE in cells, because the IgE epitope (specific fragment) against which omalizumab is targeted is already fixed to the receptors and is therefore hidden. Anti-IgE therapy is most commonly used to treat bronchial asthma but is also effective for treating allergic rhinoconjunctivitis, but therapy must begin before the pollen season [26]. The anti-IgE therapy is currently being studied for use in food allergies, but the cost has limited its use for this purpose [1].

3.3.3. *IgE blocker*

A new proposal has been studied by Deus-de-Oliveira et al. for blocking IgE-allergen binding. The identification of the IgE-binding epitopes and the amino acids involved in these interactions are fundamental steps. Deus-de-Oliveira et al. found that two glutamic acid residues in the main allergens of *Ricinus communis*, Ric c1 and Ric c 3, are involved in IgE binding, triggering an allergic response. They also found that the *Ricinus* allergens cross-reacted with aeroallergens and food allergens from several sources. Free glutamic acid can bind to castor-allergen-specific IgE, occupying the epitope-interaction site and preventing the binding of the allergens in a second exposure to the IgEs fixed in the mast cells. IgE blockade may be a safe approach for the treatment of allergy but will depend on determining the structures of allergens and on identifying epitopes and cross-allergen responses.

A summary of strategies for treating allergies is presented in **Table 3**.

Method	Advantages	Disadvantages
Antihistamines	• Alleviate the symptoms triggered by the body's responses to allergens • Effective and safe	• May cause undesirable side effects on the central nervous system • Side effects include sleepiness, sedation and fatigue that may lead to reduced cognitive, memory, and psychomotor performance
Allergen-specific immunotherapy	• Reduces the sensitivity and consequently decreases symptomatic reactions	• Specific to particular allergens
Allergen-nonspecific therapy (*anti-IgE antibodies*)	• Reduces the induced allergic responses preventing the activation of mast cells and consequently the release of allergic mediators	• Does not bind to fixed IgE in cells because the IgE epitope (specific fragment) against which omalizumab is targeted is already fixed to the receptors and is therefore masked
IgE blocker	• Blockade of IgE sites involved in the interaction with allergenic epitopes	• Under development

Table 3. Summary of strategies for treating allergies.

Author details

Olga Lima Tavares Machado*, Débora Mothé de Campos-Mesquita and Thais Pacheco-Soares

*Address all correspondence to: olga@uenf.br

Laboratory of Chemistry and Function of Proteins and Peptides, Center for Biosciences and Biotechnology, Northern State University of Rio de Janeiro - Darcy Ribeiro (CBB/UENF), Rio de Janeiro, Brazil

References

[1] Lanser BJ, Wright BL, Orgel KA, Vickery BP, Fleischer DM. Current options for the treatment of food allergy. Pediatric Clinics of North America. 2015;**62**:1531-1549

[2] D'Amato G. Role of anti-IgE monoclonal antibody (omalizumab) in the treatment of bronchial asthma and allergic respiratory diseases. European Journal of Pharmacology. 2006;**533**:302-307

[3] Larché M, Wraith DC. Peptide-based therapeutic vaccines for allergic and autoimmune diseases. Nature Medicine. 2005;**11**:S69-S76

[4] Deus-de-Oliveira N, et al. Identification of critical Amino acids in the IgE epitopes of Ric c 1 and Ric c 3 and the application of Glutamic acid as an IgE blocker. PLoS One. 2011;**6**(6):e21455

[5] Wang XY, Lim-Jurado M, Prepageran N, Tantilipikorn P, Wang DY. Treatment of allergic rhinitis and urticaria: A review of the newest antihistamine drug bilastine. Therapeutics and Clinical Risk Management. 2016;**12**:585-597

[6] Amr M Mahdy and Nigel R Webster. Histamine and antihistamines. Anaesthesia and Intensive Care Medicine. 2008;**9**:324-328

[7] Church M, Church D. Pharmacology of antihistamines. Indian Journal of Dermatology. 2013;**58**:219-224

[8] Hamilton RG, MacGlashan DW, Saini SS. IgE antibody-specific activity in human allergic disease. Immunologic Research. 2010;**47**:273-284

[9] Akdis CA, Akdis M. Mechanisms of immune tolerance to allergens: Role of IL-10 and Tregs. The Journal of clinical Investigation. 2014;**124**:4678-4680

[10] Matsuoka T, Shamji MH, Durham SR. Allergen immunotherapy and tolerance. Allergology International. 2013;**62**:403-413

[11] Jutel M, et al. Mechanisms of allergen-specific immunotherapy and novel ways for vaccine development. Allergology International. 2013;**62**:425-433

[12] Ring J, Gutermuth J. 100 years of hyposensitization: History of allergen-specific immunotherapy (ASIT). Allergy European Journal of Allergy and Clinical Immunology. 2011;**66**:713-724

[13] Holgate ST, PolosaR. Treatment strategies for allergy and asthma. Nature Reviews Immunology. 2008;**8**:218-230

[14] Kumar S., Verma A.K., Das M. , Dwivedi P. D. Molecular mechanisms of IgE mediated food allergy. International Immunopharmacology jornal. 2012;**13**:432-439

[15] Simons FER, Simons KJ. H1 antihistamines: Current status and future directions. World Allergy Organ Journal. 2008;**1**:145-155

[16] Holm J, et al. Facilitated antigen presentation and its inhibition by blocking IgG antibodies depends on IgE repertoire complexity. Journal of Allergy and Clinical. Immunology. 2011;**127**:1029-1037

[17] Geraldini M, et al. Alérgenos recombinantes na prática da imunoterapia [Recombinant allergens in immunotherapy practice]. Rev. Bras. Alergen. Imunopatol. 2008;**31**:92-97

[18] Meadows A, et al. A systematic review and economic evaluation of subcutaneous and sublingual allergen immunotherapy in adults and children with seasonal allergic rhinitis. Health Technology Assessment. 2013;**17**(27):10-19. ISSN 1366-5278

[19] Linhart B, Valenta R. Mechanisms underlying allergy vaccination with recombinant hypoallergenic allergen derivatives. Vaccine. 2012;**30**:4328-4335

[20] Valenta R, Kraft D. From allergen structure to new forms of allergen-specific immunotherapy Rudolf Valenta and Dietrich Kraft. Current Opinion in Immunology. 1991; 14718-727. DOI: 10.1016/S0952791502004028

[21] Valenta R, Campana R, Focke-Tejkl M, Niederberger V. Vaccine development for allergen-specific immunotherapy based on recombinant allergens and synthetic allergen peptides: Lessons from the past and novel mechanisms of action for the future. Journal of Allergy and Clinical Immunology. 2016;**137**:351-357

[22] Wollmann E, et al. Reduction in allergen-specific IgE binding as measured by microarray: A possible surrogate marker for effects of specific immunotherapy. Journal of Allergy and Clinical Immunology. 2015;**136**:806-809

[23] Campana R, et al. Altered IgE epitope presentation: A model for hypoallergenic activity revealed for Bet v 1 trimer. Molecular Immunology. 2011;**48**:431-441

[24] Wald M, et al. Hypoallergenic mutants of the timothy grass pollen allergen Phl p 5 generated by proline mutations. International Archives of Allergy and Immunology. 2012;**159**:130-142

[25] Campana R, et al. Frequent occurrence of T cell-mediated late reactions revealed by atopy patch testing with hypoallergenic rBet v 1 fragments. Journal of Allergy and Clinical Immunology. 2016;**137**:601-609

[26] Blank U, Charles N, Benhamou M. The high-affinity immunoglobulin e receptor as pharmacological target. European Journal of Pharmacology. 2016;**778**:24-32

[27] Nowak-we A, Sampson HA. Future therapies for food allergies. 2011;**127**:558-573. DOI: 10.1016/j.jaci.2010.12.1098

Chapter 5

Allergen-Based Diagnostic: Novel and Old Methodologies with New Approaches

Alberto Salazar, Henry Velázquez-Soto,
Julio Ayala-Balboa and María C. Jiménez-Martínez

Additional information is available at the end of the chapter

http://dx.doi.org/10.5772/intechopen.69276

Abstract

This chapter is an extensive review of allergen-based diagnostic methodologies including old techniques such as skin prick test, radio-allergo sorbent test, enzyme-linked immunosorbent assay, and fluorescent-enzyme immunosorbent assay. Novel technologies include functional tests by flow cytometry and molecular allergy based on multiplex immunoassays. We also review the importance of biochemical characteristics of allergens, sensitivity and specificity, cross-reaction between allergens, utility, reproducibility, interpretation, and methodologies for discovery of epitopes for diagnostic or therapeutic use.

Keywords: allergens, skin prick test, RAST, ELISA, FEIA, ISAC, FACS, BAT, flow cytometry, antigen-antibody reaction, diagnostic

1. Introduction

Allergic diseases have been considered a worldwide health problem. The incidence and prevalence of hypersensitivity/allergy conditions are increasing every day, affecting people of any age, damaging a broad range of organs, and making a diagnostic challenge for the clinician [1]. It is well known that an accurate diagnosis could affect the clinical outcome; this is particularly important for the treatment of allergic diseases because the identification of the causative antigen and other molecules associated with specific immunological activation by allergen-based tests allows personalized medicine and precision treatment [2].

2. Historical perspective of allergen-based diagnostic methodologies

2.1. Skin prick test (SPT)

Skin prick testing is an essential clinical test to confirm sensitization in IgE-mediated allergic diseases. Historically, we can found an early report in 1850, in a textbook of Henry Salter, a physician from London´s Charing Cross Hospital who described the formation of wheals following scratches in patients with asthma and exposed to cats [3]. In 1907, Clemens von Pirquet reported a modification of Koch´s subcutaneous procedure based in abrasion of the skin to evaluate tuberculin response [4]. This procedure was rapidly adopted by others as a prototype for prick-puncture testing, and in 1909, the first case of anaphylactic response after scarification and exposition to an allergen was reported [5]. Practical application of a standardized procedure was suggested by Schloss [6] who described a correlation of time with clinical signs, reporting 5–15 min of erythematous reaction after abrasion of the skin in a child with rhinitis, asthma, and eczema. Since then, several techniques to evaluate allergenic sensitization have been described, e.g., intracutaneous test, [7] conjunctival test, [8] intracutaneous test by serial dilutions [9]. Nowadays the best technique to evaluate with safety allergenic sensitization is the SPT.

The standardized method of prick testing includes the appropriate selection of allergens, i.e., allergens tested are according to the country, the geographic location inside the same country, and even with seasons [10, 11]. SPT is based on the presence of sensitized cells, mainly mast cells in the skin, and the resulted cutaneous reactivity is used by the clinician as a surrogate biomarker for sensitization in eyes, nose, lung, gut, and skin. During the test, positive and negative controls must be included, a positive result is defined with a wheal ≥3 mm diameter after 15–20 min; reproducible results are obtained with standardized mixtures [12, 13]. In the early years of use, skin prick testing did not have with the entire approbation of the medical community, and their clinical relevance was questioned [14]. That vision has changed, and in the last years, it has been recognized a concordance between the clinical manifestations and allergen-specific wheal size [15]. Thus, skin prick test is considered as a fundamental technique to explore allergen sensitization in patients, but if it is true, why we need other methods to study sensitization in allergic/hypersensitivity conditions? In the following paragraphs, we will explain applications of the most common laboratory assays used to evaluate IgE specificity and the information obtained in functional allergen-based tests.

2.2. IgE and allergy

The discovery of the reaginic activity in the IgE antibody by Ishizaka in 1967 [16] developed a revolution in the knowledge of allergy affecting not only in basic research but also in applied research resulting in innovative diagnostic tools. It is well known that patients with allergy have a tendency to produce high levels of IgE antibodies due to its atopic condition. Usually, the concentration of total IgE in serum from healthy individuals ranges below 1 μg/mL. It is worthy of note that this is a very low concentration of protein so many laboratories rather use IU/mL or kU/L instead of μg/mL to report IgE levels, but understanding that 1 kU/L equals to 2.4 ng/mL [17]. Total IgE does not correlate with clinical manifestations, and is preferably to measure specific IgE (sIgE) [18, 19]. Total IgE concentration is the addition of all the specific IgE (sIgE) to the different allergens the individual has been exposed to; in non-allergic subjects, sIgE levels are below the limits of detection (0.35 kU/L) [20]. Thus, to identify the triggering antigen of allergic manifestations, one of the most common laboratory test requirement is the determination of sIgE concentration in serum. The quantification of sIgE can be performed through several methods based on antigen-antibody reaction, e.g., radio allergo sorbent test (RAST), enzyme-linked immunosorbent assay (ELISA) and fluorescence enzyme immune assay (FEIA).

3. Antigen-antibody reaction for IgE detection: general principle

Quantification of IgE is based on the antigen-antibody reaction, in which antigen is recognized specifically by an antibody forming an immune complex (**Figure 1**). In these tests, the antigen corresponds to serum IgE, and the antibody reacts against IgE in the serum sample. To carry out these assays, a specific antibody for the Fc fraction of the IgE is adsorbed into a solid phase usually in polystyrene or cellulose wells. This so-called "primary antibody" or "capture antibody" has the function of binding to the IgE in the sample of serum; this interaction generates a stable bound. Then, this immune complex is measured through a second antibody called "secondary antibody" or "detection antibody" which is coupled to a radioisotope (RAST) or an enzyme which allows the development of a colored (ELISA) or fluorescent (FEIA) substrate in an antigen-dependent manner. Simultaneously, a calibration curve containing known concentrations of the analyte to determine is processed to extrapolate the data of absorbance (in colorimetric methods—ELISA) or the fluorescence (in fluorometric methods—FEIA) to a protein concentration, finally reported in µg, ng, or IU.

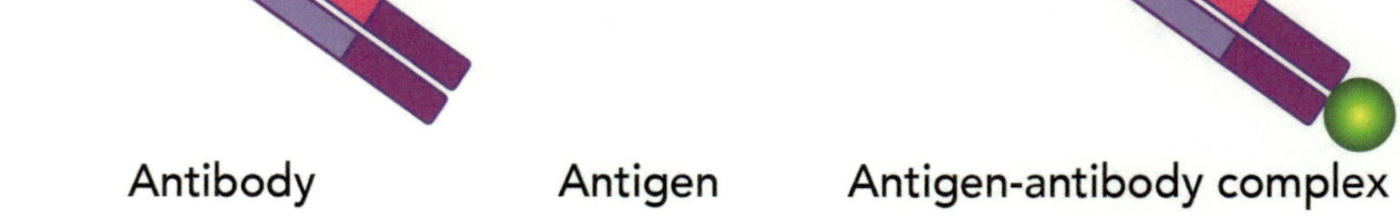

Figure 1. Antigen-antibody reaction. Each antibody is able to bind its specific antigen, forming antigen-antibody complexes. Different laboratory testing techniques are based on this principle.

3.1. Radio allergo sorbent test (RAST)

RAST was the first laboratory method developed for *in vitro* detection of specific IgE [21]; despite that it is no longer used and its historical importance is evident since it was the second most used test after SPT, and gave rise to development of new methodology to facilitate sIgE detection. The main advantage of this method over SPT lied on the safety of patient. In SPT, the allergen is administered in the cutaneous layer of the skin, which may lead to sensitization to new allergens or in the worst of cases it may trigger anaphylaxis. All of the previous disadvantages were avoided with the introduction of *in vitro* tests like RAST.

As mentioned above, this test is based on the principle of antigen-antibody reaction. In this method, the allergen is adsorbed covalently to a solid particle, then, the serum of a patient is added. IgE antibodies present in the sample binds to the adsorbed allergen. After this, a washing step is needed to remove non-specific weak bindings. Next, a radio-iodinated anti-IgE antibody is added to this reaction, and finally, the radiation detected is directly proportional to the number of antigen-antibody complexes formed (**Figure 2**).

This method was validated in comparison with sIgE in pollen-sensitized individuals, finding 96% of concordance with both tests [22].

3.2. Enzyme-linked immunosorbent assay (ELISA)

ELISA is currently one of the most common immune-assays used in clinical and experimental procedures. This technique allows detection of allergy-related analytes, e.g., IgE or Th2 cytokines, and screening of different molecules. Advantages of ELISA are fast performance, improved biosafety when compared with radioimmunoassay, low reagent cost, affordability for the patient, and simple methodology [23].

The first step to perform an ELISA is sensitizing the plate. A solid polystyrene plate is coated with an anti-IgE antibody directed against Fc region of the immunoglobulin (capture antibody). This process is achieved pre-treating the plate wells with carbonate buffers or cyanogen bromide allowing a better chance for adsorbing the capture antibody or antigen. Another

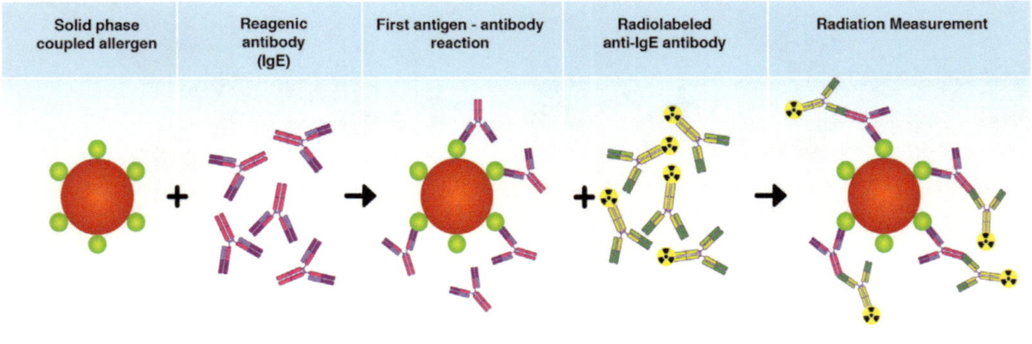

Figure 2. RAST methodology. An allergen is adsorbed covalently to a solid particle, then serum of patient is added to react with the allergen. Next, a radiolabeled anti-IgE antibody identifies the previous formed immune complexes. The radiation generated is measured by a radiation detector.

http://dx.doi.org/10.5772/intechopen.69276

strategy is to radiate the polystyrene plate; this permits the breaking of a certain number of benzene rings yielding carboxyl (COOH) and hydroxyl (OH) groups. Radiation of polystyrene increases the chances for hydrophilic interactions with Fc fractions of capture antibody. Protein A from *Staphylococcus aureus* is also a suitable linker for orienting and spacing the capture antibody appropriately, optimizing the space, and homogenizing the coating. In this step, several factors like pH and temperature could affect the proper adsorption of antibody or allergen. Fortunately, commercial kits contain the pre-sensitized plates. Next step is incubation of samples (serum or plasma), although serum samples are preferred over plasma samples since some commercial houses have documented diminishing IgE detection sensitivity in plasma samples.

Incubation let the captured antibody bind to IgE through Fc fraction (in total IgE determination) or allows the specific IgE contained in the sample bind to the allergen adsorbed in the solid phase (in specific IgE determination). After incubation time, a washing step is performed to remove weak and unspecific binding. Then, a second anti-Fc antibody is added to the well to detect the immune complexes formed in the previous step. This "secondary or detection antibody" is linked to an oxidative enzyme that acts on its substrate which once oxidized develops a color that can be measured trough a spectrophotometer (**Figure 3**).

There are various enzymes and substrates commonly used in ELISA (**Table 1**); the biotin-streptavidin system is the most often employed in detection methods. A washing step is followed next to eliminate the excess of not bound antibodies. In addition to samples, control or standard curve is processed with increasing concentrations of protein. The goal of this standard curve is to extrapolate the absorbance obtained from samples into a curve of known concentration through a linear regression, and obtaining an estimated concentration of the analyte (**Figure 4**).

The last step consists in adding and incubating the substrate for 10–20 min and reading the absorbance obtained after stopping the reaction. Some substrates may be read without stopping

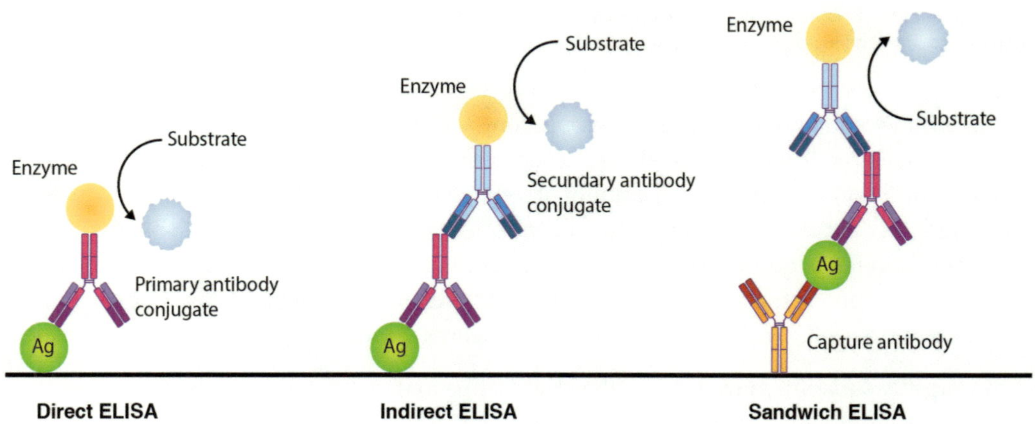

Figure 3. ELISA assays. Direct ELISA mostly used for antigen detection. Indirect ELISA mainly used for antibodies detection. Sandwich ELISA used to detect total IgE.

Enzyme	Substrate	Wavelength after stop solution (nm)
Horse radish peroxidase (HRP)	3,3′,5,5′-tetramethylbenzidine, TMB	450
	2,2′-Azinobis (3-Ethylenbenzothiazoline-6-sulfonic acid) diamonium salt, ABTS	450
	o-phenylenediamine dyhidocloride, OPD	490
Alkaline phosphatase (AP)	p-Nitrophenyl phospate disodium salt	450

Table 1. Enzymes and substrates used in ELISA assays.

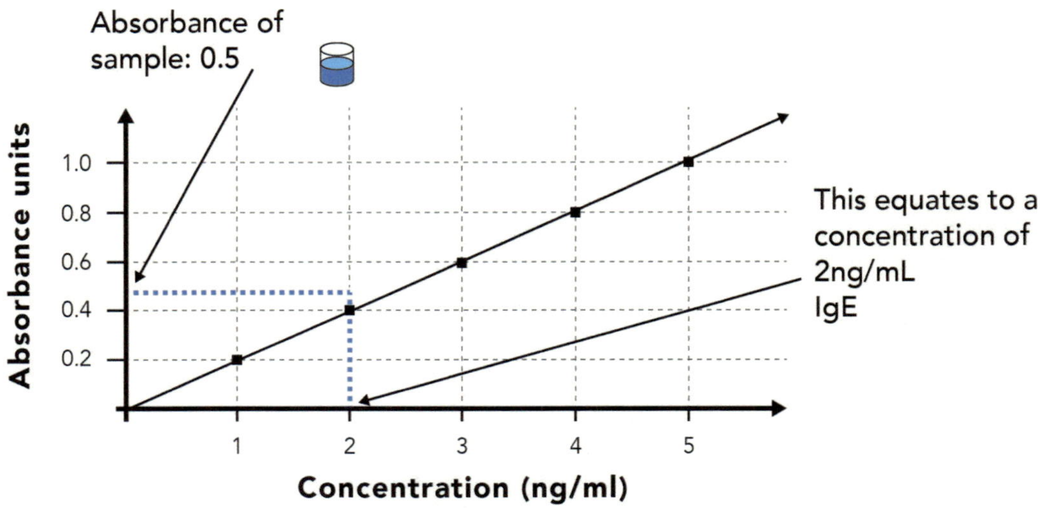

Figure 4. Absorbance-concentration standard curve. In order to determine sIgE concentration in a sample, a standard curve is run using known concentrations of total or allergen-specific IgE. By plotting the absorbance from patient samples into the standard curve, we can determine sIgE concentration.

the reaction. Results are read in a spectrophotometer; this equipment works emitting a light beam that is filtered through a wavelength selector or filter; then, the filtered light will strike the sample, which will absorb a certain amount of light and let some light pass and reach the detector. Absorbance is the negative logarithm of transmittance, so the absorbance obtained will be proportional to the concentration of the measured antigen-antibody complexes in the samples that may reflect and refract the light at a certain wavelength (**Figure 5**). Optical density (OD) is a common term used to refer to absorbance (see **Figures 4** and **5**).

ELISA rapidly substituted radiolabeled methods, due to its safer and faster performance, with a similar sensibility and specificity when compared to RAST and paper radio immuno-sorbent test (PRIST) for total or specific IgE quantification [24, 25].

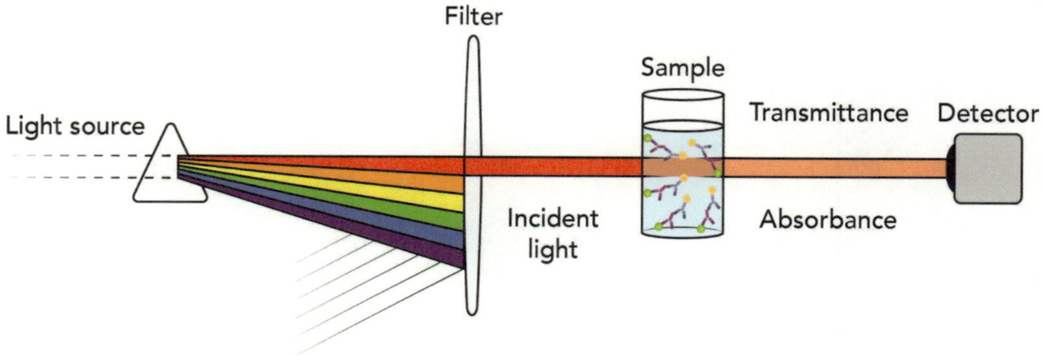

Figure 5. Spectrophotometer basis. A light beam is generated by a halogen lamp, and this light is filtered through a wavelength selector. Light hits the sample and the transmittance measured is reported as absorbance units. Absorbance is directly proportional to the amount of antibody-antigen complexes formed previously.

3.3. Fluorescent enzyme immune assay (FEIA)

Fluorescent enzyme immune assays are based on the same principle used for ELISA and RAST, the antigen-antibody reaction, but differs in the way the read out is made. In FEIA, the secondary antibody is linked to an enzyme that permits the activation of a fluorochrome. The most common enzyme used in fluorometric assays is β-galactosidase, which acts on its substrate 4-methylumbelliferyl-β-D-galactoside transforming it into a 4-methylumbelliferone. When 4-methylumbelliferone is excited at 365 nm, it emits fluorescence at 445 nm. This fluorescence is later measured by a fluorometer [26]. Simultaneously, a standard curve is processed to extrapolate the relative fluorescence units obtained from samples into the known concentration curve (**Figure 6**).

Fluorometric assays have permitted the development of automatized systems, resulting in improved reproducibility, diminished operator involvement, with reduction of mistakes, and increased sensitivity and specificity when compared with other innovative methods based on chemiluminescence [27, 28]. FEIA technology opens the possibility to screen sIgE to several allergens at the same time and with few volume of sample [29]. **Table 2** shows a comparison between antigen-antibody reaction-based methods for quantification of sIgE.

3.4. ImmunoCAP-ISAC (immuno solid-phase allergen chip)

Innovative and non-invasive techniques led to the identification of many sIgE to different allergens at the same time, with a minimum sample volume (~50 μL), allowing test allergens not limited to a geographical region, and without risk of sensitization, or anaphylaxis for the patient, as has been reported for SPT [30].

ISAC is the first multiplex diagnostic tool commercially available to evaluate sIgE directed against 112 well-characterized antigens. In fact, the allergens presented in the solid phase are recombinant proteins ensuring specific interaction of serum IgE with higher accuracy when

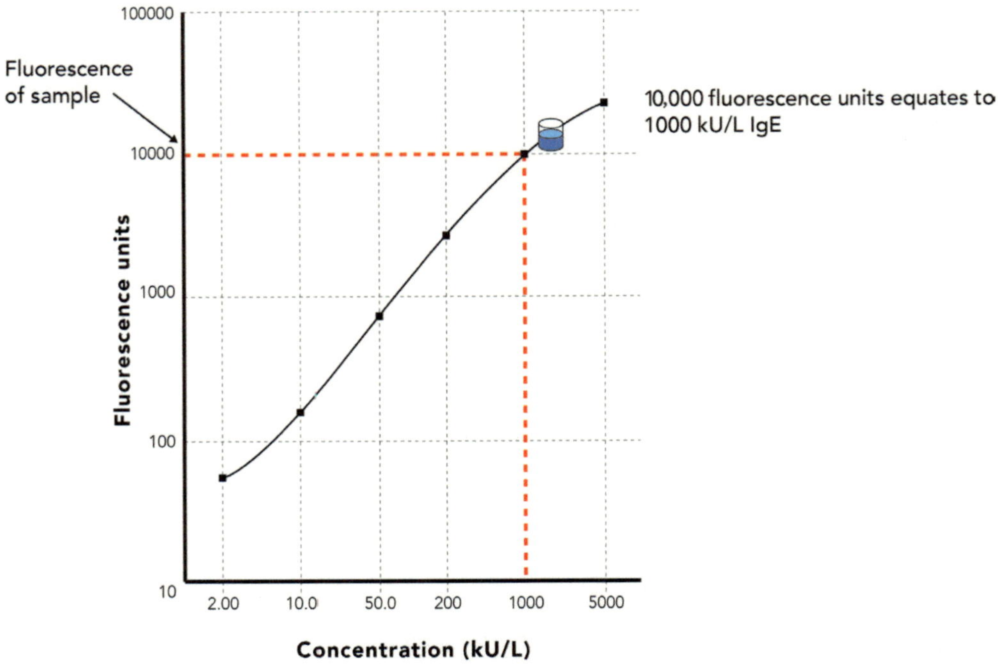

Figure 6. Fluorescence-concentration standard curve. Quantification of sIgE is measured plotting fluorescence units obtained from samples into a standard curve.

Test	RAST	ELISA	FEIA
Specificity	Depends on antigen preparation	High	High
Sensitivity	High	High	High
Reproducibility	Acceptable	Acceptable	High
Automatization	Partially	Partially	Totally
Relative cost per test	Low	Affordable	High
Shelf life of reagents	Long	Low	Long
Health hazards for laboratory personnel	High	Non or minor	Non or minor

Table 2. Methods for sIgE quantification based on the antigen-antibody reaction.

compared with FEIA and SPT [31]. The assay consists of various steps. First, the sIgE from serum samples interacts with the recombinant allergen previously adsorbed to the solid-phase; then, a secondary anti-human IgE antibody labeled with fluorochrome recognizes sIgE-recombinant allergen complex (**Figure 7**). Fluorescence is measured using a biochip; and results are scanned and analyzed in specialized software, reporting results in arbitrary units named ISAC Standardized Units (ISU) (**Figure 8**) [32].

http://dx.doi.org/10.5772/intechopen.69276

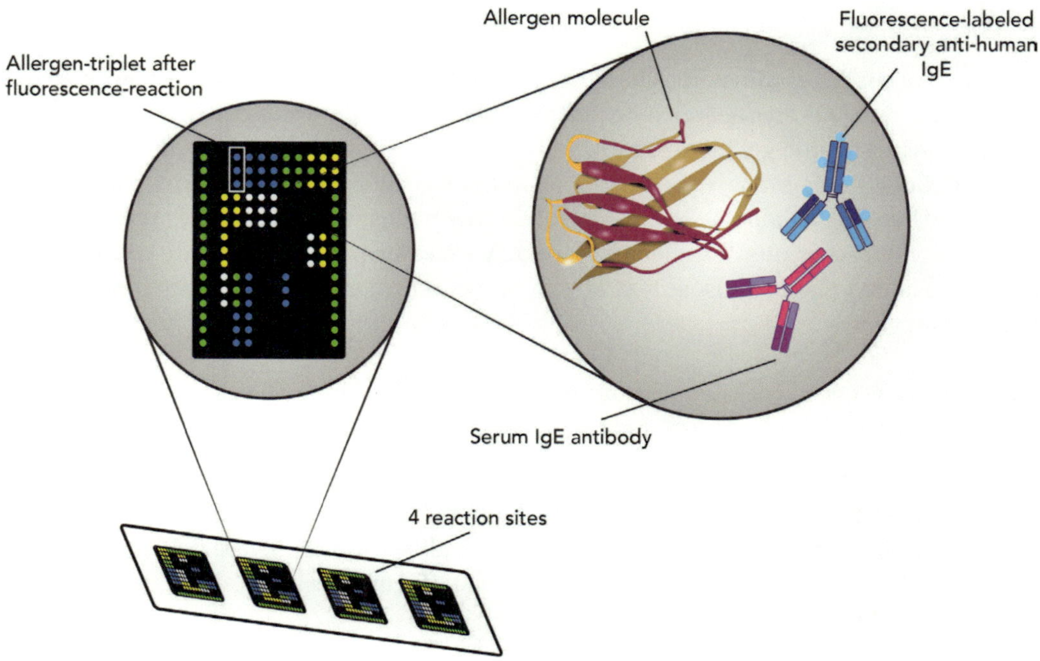

Figure 7. Immuno CAP-ISAC. The recombinant allergens are recognized by sIgE from serum samples; a secondary antibody fluorescent-labeled interacts with IgE. Fluorescence is measured by a biochip and results are analyzed in specialized software. Recombinant allergen diminishes the risk of cross-reactivity.

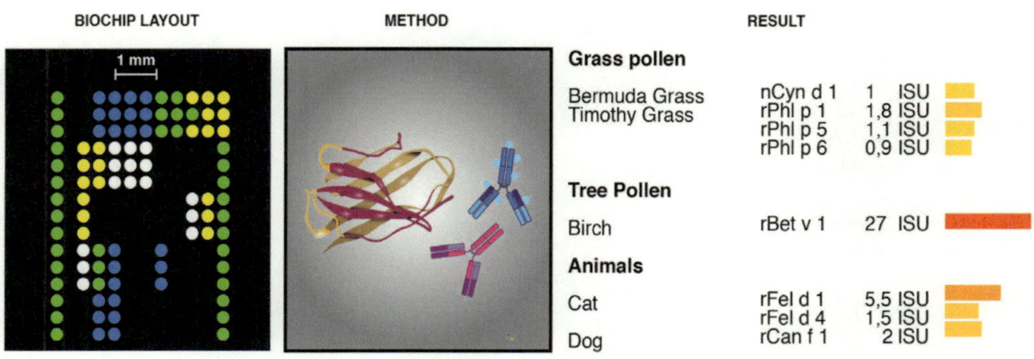

Figure 8. ISAC biochip layout. Results are reported in arbitrary units named ISAC-Standardized Units (ISU).

ISAC multiplex assay has been proposed to guide therapeutic decisions, e.g., the discontinuation of restrictive diets, the content of allergen-specific desensitization immunotherapy that may be useful to discriminate structurally similar allergens and cross-reactivity, and even to analyze the real sensitization profile in multi-sensitized patients to define whether they can receive a specific immunotherapy [33].

3.5. Western blot

Western blot combines different techniques to identify new antigens related to allergy. In this method, the antigens are separated according to their molecular weight in a sodium dodecyl sulfate polyacrylamide gel (SDS-PAGE), and then transferred to a polyvinylidene difluoride or nitrocellulose membrane, which will function as the solid phase for the antigen-antibody reaction. Then, the membrane is incubated with the patient serum, if sIgE is present in the sample it will react against the allergens found. A secondary anti-IgE antibody coupled to an enzyme is added (**Table 1**). Detection of sIgE becomes evident by the formation of bands in two different ways:

(a) Developing color. The enzyme oxidizes the substrate and precipitates (e.g., when using a secondary antibody conjugated to horse radish peroxidase (HRP) and 4-cloronaphthol).

(b) Releasing light. The substrate is dephosphorylated by an enzyme, releasing light (chemiluminescence), that is later detected by a photographic film or autoradiography (i.e., when using a secondary antibody conjugated to alkaline phosphatase (AP) and adamantyl-1,2-dioxetane phosphate or HRP and luminol) (**Figure 9**). Finally, concentration can be estimated by densitometer analysis.

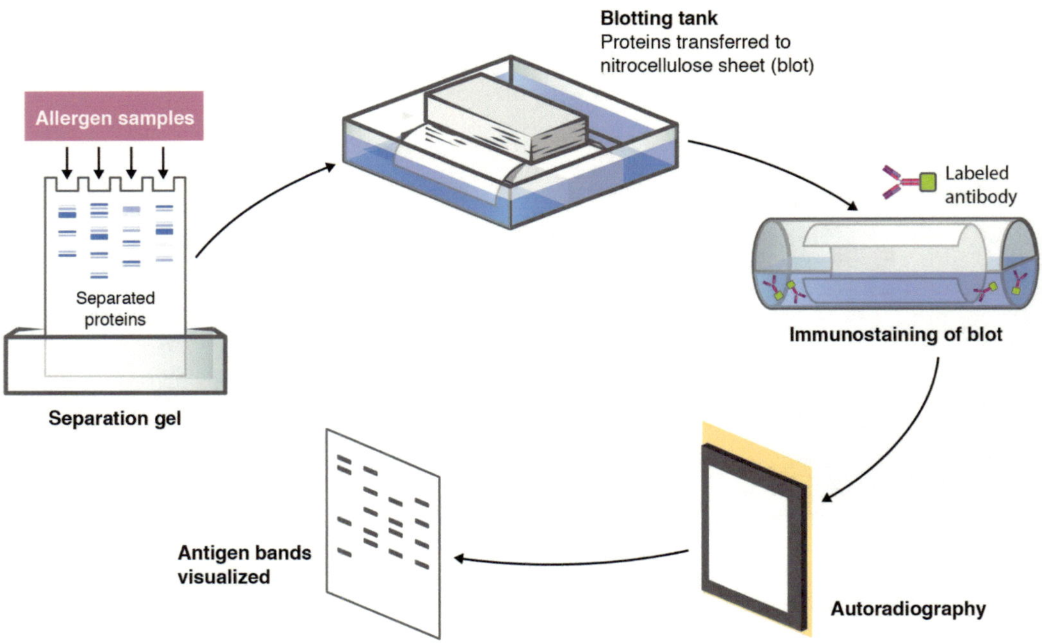

Figure 9. Western-blot methodology. Allergen mixtures are separated in a SDS-PAGE according to the molecular size. The separated allergens are transferred to a nitrocellulose or PVDF membrane. Then, by adding the antibodies from the serum samples sIgE will bind to their specific antigen. An enzyme conjugate secondary antibody identifies Fcε IgE. Detection of reaginic antibodies is identified by chemiluminescence.

This method has been useful in the identification of clinically relevant immunogenic epitopes after enzymatic digestion of allergens and is also used to identify cross-reacting peptides [34–36].

4. Limitations of sIgE determinations: allergen cross-reactivity

Something to consider when handling sIgE quantification is the cross-reactivity of certain allergens. Some allergens share amino acidic sequences that can be recognized by the same IgE antibody, and this phenomenon is called "cross-reactivity." Cross-reactivity occurs mainly in aeroallergens and food allergens. It is considered to have a high chance of cross-reactivity when two allergens share 35% homology in an 80-amino acid sequence or full identity in a 6–8 amino acid peptide; also, there may be a cross-reaction when the IgE is specific for carbohydrate moiety in the allergen. Hence, laboratory blood tests may detect antibodies to allergens even if the patient has never been exposed to them [37].

Importantly cross-reactivity can occur between allergens from the same family like in nut allergens or in different species of house dust mite; but also, cross-reactivity could be present in diverse phylogenetic sources like house dust mite and shrimp, birch and apple, or fish and chicken meat (**Table 3**) [38–40]. As we read in the previous section, technology innovation through recombinant allergens and full automatization notably reduce cross-reactivity risk when performing sIgE determinations.

Cross-reactivity	***Antigens* involved on cross-reactivity**
Birch-apple	Bet v1 homologue Mal d1
Cypress-peach	Pru p3 non-specific lipid transfer protein (LTP)
Celery-mugwort-spice	Art v4 profilin, Art v60 kDa homologue to Api g5
Mugwort-peach	Art v4 profilin, Art v3 LTP
Alternaria-spinach	Alt a1
Mite-shrimp	Der p10, tropomyosin
Cat-pork	Fel d2 cat serum albumin
Bird-egg	Gal d5 alpha-livetin (chicken serum albumin)

Table 3. Allergen cross-reactivity and antigens involved.

5. Functional tests

The techniques above described answer two simple requests: is the sIgE present in the sample? So, if there, how much sIgE is present? The answer to these questions and the analysis of the clinical history allows the allergist/immunologist to initiate treatments centered on allergen-specific desensitization in every single patient in a personalized way. However, sometimes answer to these questions is not enough, and functional tests are needed to understand some clinical manifestations, e.g. allergy to a particular drug.

5.1. Flow cytometry and fluorescence-activated cell sorting (FACS)

Early in the 1950s, Coulter developed a technology able to read size and complexity of blood cells based on diffraction of light laying the fundamentals for automatized blood counting used in our days. Exploiting this innovation, Bonner, Sweet, Hulett, Herzenberg invented the Fluorescence Activated Cell Sorter (FACS) in the late 1960s to achieve flow cytometry and cell sorting of viable cells. Becton Dickinson with Bernie Shoor introduced the commercial cytometers in the early 1970s, utilizing a Stanford patent and the expertise supplied by the Herzenberg Laboratory [41]. Today, isolation of cells by FACS is performed in complete sterility, and sorted cells could be used as an adoptive transfer for therapeutical interventions [42].

Flow cytometry detects and analyzes optical signals (angular light scatter or emitted fluorescence) to identify individual characteristics of cells or in biological samples. Inside the flow cytometer, the suspended cells are conducted in a fluidic system ensuring cells travel at a uniform velocity in a laminar form. Here, the cells are directed to a specific point in which a laser passes through cells. The light is diffracted in all directions, the emitted light is recovered in filters, and photodetectors collect the detection signals. The optical detection system obtains information about forward light scatter (FSC), side light scatter (SSC), and fluorescence channels (FL1, FL2, FL3). Then, the luminous signal is detected in photomultiplier tubes; information recollected is digitalized that is to be analyzed by a computer system. Information obtained is showed in histograms or dot plots. The quality of both systems (optical and fluidic) is critical for performance and reliability of this technique [43] (**Figure 10**).

Flow cytometry could be used to determine the expression of cell surface markers, to know absolute or relative numbers of cells, to determine intracellular proteins, to quantify soluble proteins, or combine all of these possibilities.

(a) Expression of cell surface markers. Information obtained by analysis of expression of cell surface markers could be useful to know the cellular phenotype and some functions of labeled cells. A few examples include the state of activation of a particular cell [e.g., CD63 on basophils after drug exposition (see the next section of this chapter for a deeper explanation of basophils activation test)], to know absolute numbers of circulating cells (e.g., 1700 CD4/μL), or combining information (e.g., patients with ocular allergy have increasing percentage of circulating helper activated CD4+CD25+ T cells) [44].

(b) Determination of intracellular proteins. This procedure is useful to assess specific functions of the cell. First, isolation of cells is needed prior incubation with a stimulus (e.g., allergens as specific stimulus). Culture or incubation conditions must be standardized to ensure reproducibility of results. It is important to note that if studied protein is secreted (e.g., cytokines) protein secretion must be inhibited (e.g., brefeldin-A that blocks internal protein transport) to allow retention of proteins inside the cytoplasm. Labeling of intracellular proteins is performed after cells were fixed and permeabilized with detergents (e.g.,

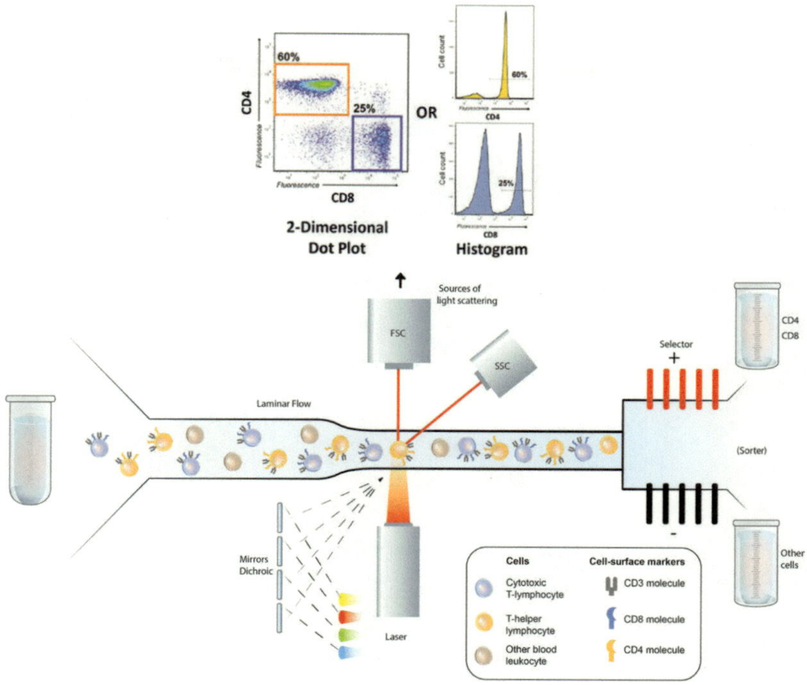

Figure 10. Flow cytometer and fluorescent activated cell sorter. The figure resumes the optical and the fluidic systems working together to analyze biophysical characteristics of cells, expression of molecules detected by monoclonal antibodies, and sorting of cells expressing selected characteristics.

saponin). Permeabilization process ensures that monoclonal antibodies (mAbs) labeled with fluorochromes enter into the cell and react with their specific antigens (**Figure 11**) [45]. The determination of intracellular proteins has significantly contributed to the understanding of physiopathology induced by allergens (e.g., Allergen-activation induces cytokines related to the damage of IL-25 in asthma, IL-31 in atopic dermatitis, and IL-5 in vernal conjunctivitis) [46–48].

(c) Quantification of soluble proteins. The determination of soluble proteins could be used to know normal ranges of proteins in human fluids or to assess cellular functions. Multiplex technology has been developed to detect several proteins in the same sample, and it is named cytometric bead arrays (CBA). The advantage of this test is the low volume of sample letting to process a broad range of human fluids/secretions (e.g., tears, synovial fluid, aqueous humor, and serum) and cell supernatants [49–52].

Multiple determinations of soluble proteins by flow cytometry are based in microspheres, all of them conjugated with a specific antibody against protein we wish to determine. After bead interacts with its antigen, a second antibody labeled with a fluorochrome is added; usually, this secondary antibody is conjugated to phycoerythrine (PE). However, the real innovation of this assay is that each bead is also labeled with a different fluorochrome in a range of intensity, from low intensity to high intensity, and detected by near infrared (NIR) lasers [53, 54] (**Figure 12**).

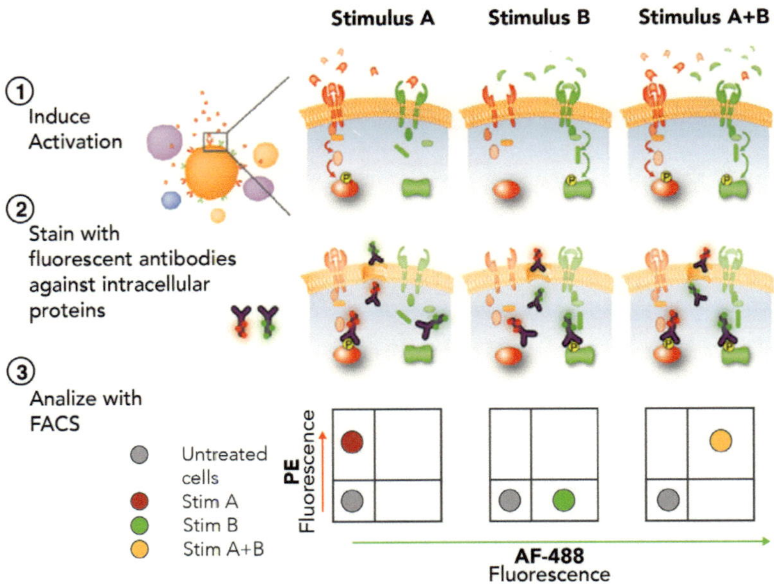

Figure 11. Determination of intracellular proteins by flow cytometry. Identification of intracellular proteins allows studying cellular functions.

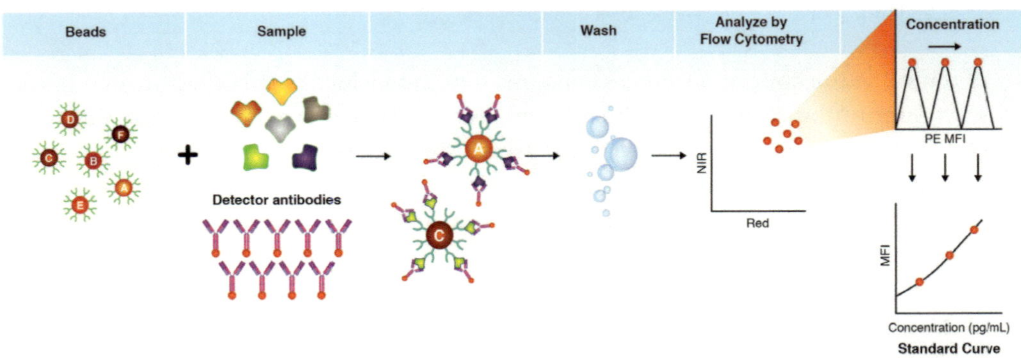

Figure 12. Cytometric bead arrays. Multiplex technology permits determination of various soluble proteins at the same time, and in the same sample.

Changes in intensity of fluorescence are expressed as median fluorescence intensity (MFI) and directly correlate with concentration of protein in the sample expressed in pg/mL or ng/mL (**Figure 13**).

5.1.1. Basophils activation test (BAT)

Adverse drug reactions (ADR) constitute a major health problem worldwide with high morbidity and mortality rates, the incidence of fatal ADR occurs in 5% in hospitalized patients in Europe [55]. ADR may be classified as Type A (augmentation of normal drug effects), Type B

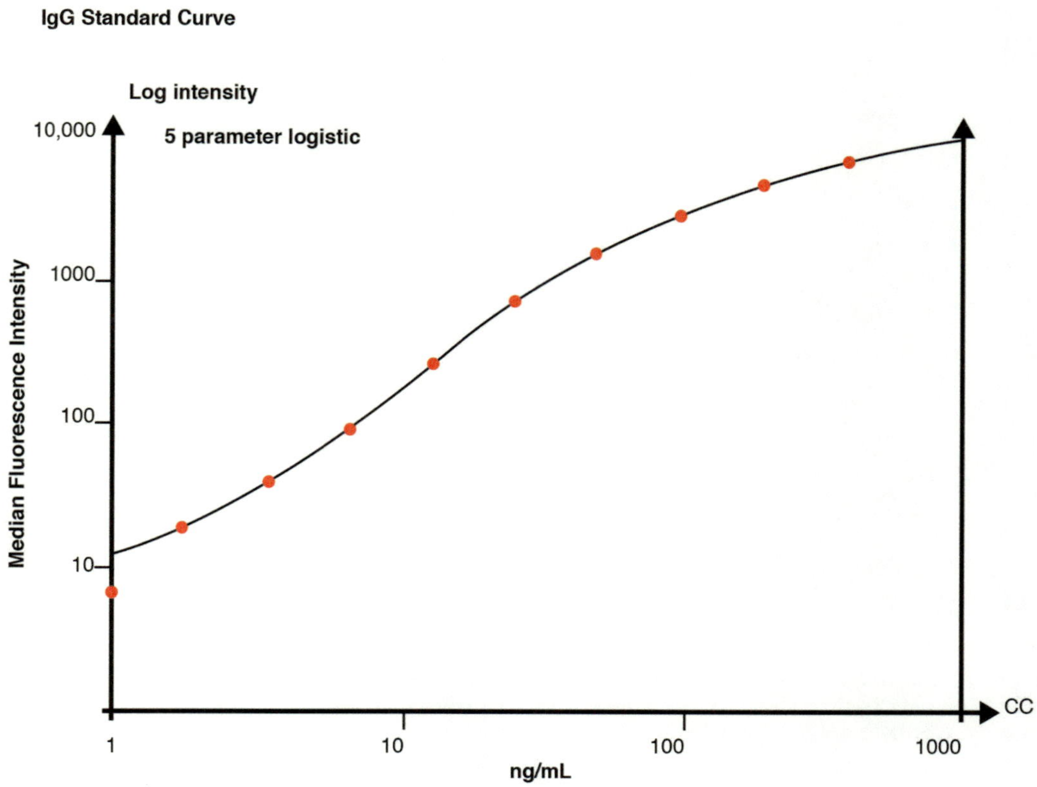

Figure 13. Standard-curve and median fluorescence intensity (MFI). Changes in MFI correlate with concentration of soluble protein.

(bizarre effects), Type C (chronic effects), Type D (delayed effects), and Type E (end of drug use effects). The most frequent ADR are Type A and are related to genetics, age, sex, and disease, and they have low mortality and high morbidity; in contrast, Type B are 25% of ADR and are unpredictable, with high mortality and low morbidity. The pathophysiological mechanisms of Type B reactions are not well understood. Some cases are mediated by type I hypersensitivity (true allergy), but other cases are related with the generation of reactive metabolites that react non-enzymatically on multiple proteins to form immunogenic-drugs complexes that induce a cascade of cell-based reactions and result in a wide range of severe clinical symptoms [56]. Due to the complexity of ADR, only Type B reactions could be explored by basophil activation test (BAT).

Principle of this test is simple, basophils are activated *in vitro* by the suspicious drug; if basophils are sensitized to the drug, they become active, upregulating on their surface two molecules CD63 and CD203c [57]. CD63 is an intracellular lysosomal protein whose surface expression is upregulated after activation. CD63 is also expressed on activated platelets, degranulated neutrophils, monocytes, macrophages, and endothelium [58]. On the other hand, CD203c is an ectoenzyme located both on the plasma membrane and in the cytoplasmic compartment of basophils. Cross-linking of the FcεRI by an allergen or anti-IgE antibody results in a rapid upregulation of intracellular CD203c molecules to the cell surface and is accompanied by mediator release [59] (**Figure 14**).

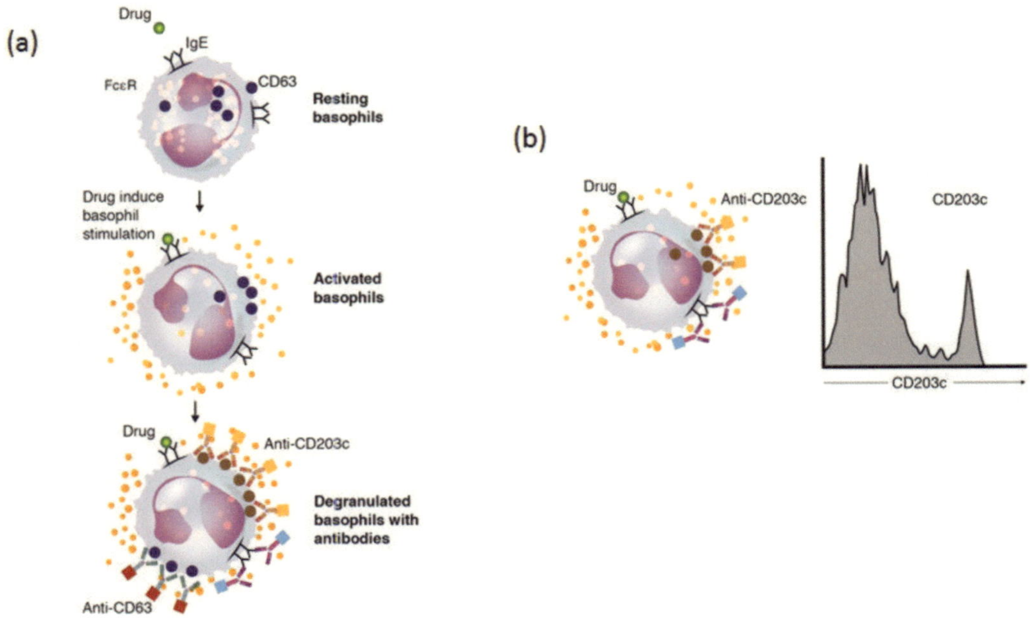

Figure 14. Basophils activation test. (a) After activation basophils upregulate CD63 and CD203c on membrane surface. Both CD63 and CD203c are detected by antibodies conjugated to fluorochromes; (b) the histogram shows increased expression of CD203c on gated basophils.

Reports about sensitivity and specificity for BAT indicate that determination of both, CD63 and CD203c, considerably increases the sensitivity up to 92% and specificity in a range of 86–90% [60, 61]. Today, BAT is also used to determine sensitization to several allergens such as diverse types of pollen and house dust mites. It has been reported that BAT has the same sensitivity but lower specificity when compared with FEIA. BAT could be used as an alternative to SPT in some patients with allergy to aeroallergens [62] and as a useful test preventing preoperative anaphylaxis [63].

BAT assay is performed with 100 μL of peripheral blood; the drug is incubated with the blood at 1 mg/mL, in 36.5°C of temperature and atmosphere of 5% CO_2 during 1 h; as an internal control, the same volume of blood is incubated with negative or positive controls. N-formyl-methionyl-leucyl-phenylalanine (f-MLP) is used as positive control. f-MLP is an N-formylated tripeptide that functions as a chemotactic peptide for polymorphonuclear (PMN) cells but is a potent activator of basophils too. After incubation, cells are labeled with monoclonal antibodies for 30 min, and then erythrocytes are lysed and results are analyzed by flow cytometry. To ensure that CD63 expressing cells are basophils, analyzed cells are also labeled against CD123 and Human leukocyte antigen-DR (HLA-DR). CD123 is the IL-3Rα, granulocytes including basophils, that constitutively express this cluster of differentiation [64]; whereas HLA-DR is expressed on B lymphocytes, monocytes, macrophages, activated T lymphocytes, activated natural killer (NK) lymphocytes but is absent in basophils. First, we analyzed cells by their complexity (SSC) and expression of CD123 and HLA-DR, basophils would be CD123+HLA-DR−, and only if activated by allergen or drug-medication, basophils would be CD63+ CD203c+ (SSC/CD123+HLA-DR−CD63+CD203c+) (**Figure 15**).

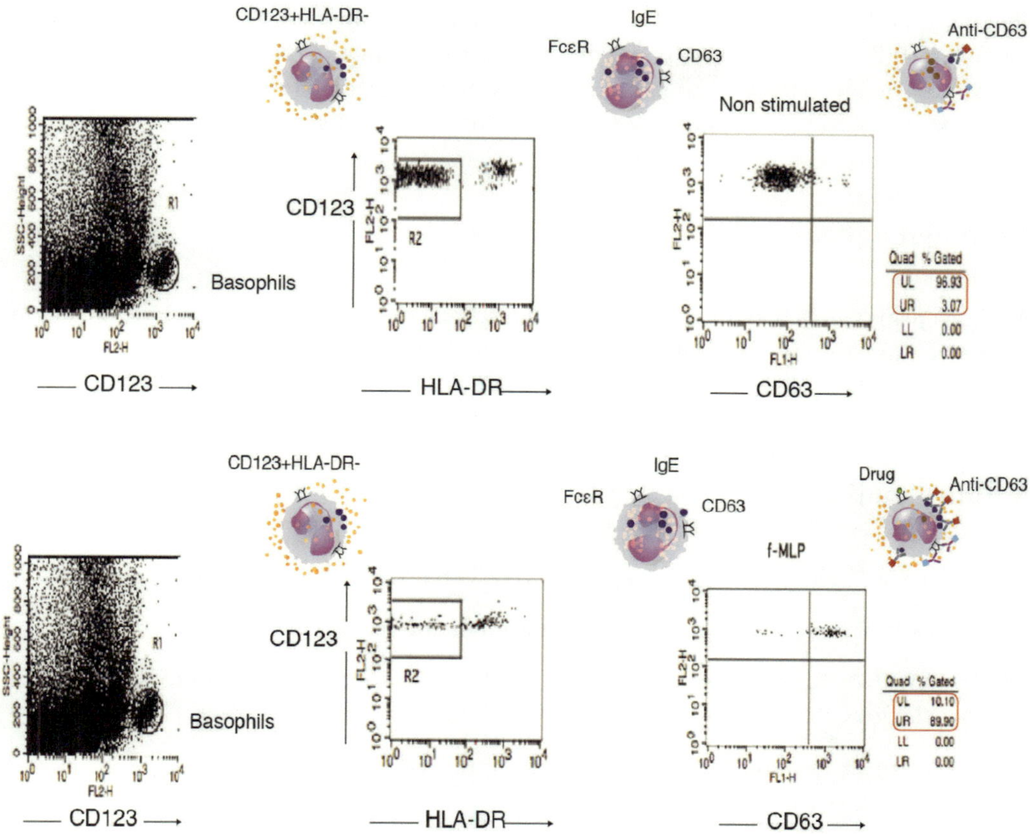

Figure 15. Representative dot plot of flow cytometry analysis of a basophils activated test. Upper panel shows non-stimulated cells. The lower panel shows stimulated cells with f-MLP. Percentage of activated basophils is showed at the squares next to dot plots.

6. Conclusions

The analytical and functional methods described in this chapter are evolved significantly since the first clinical report related to the identification of a triggering allergen in an asthmatic patient. All the allergen-based diagnostic methodologies revised in this chapter are grounded in the antigen-antibody reaction; recognizing the advantages and disadvantages of each analytic method is essential to make adequate choices. Although the apparent simplicity of methods is described here, some technical considerations have to be considered to avoid human errors when performing and interpreting sIgE tests.

It is important to note that the understanding of these techniques could be easy, but to apply them to make therapeutical decisions is not as easy. Allergic diseases are the best example of precision medicine. In this context, the therapeutical interventions through allergen-specific desensitization and addition of biologicals to block the function of certain molecules must be argued not only with evidence-based medicine but also with a personalized analysis of every single patient. Today technology is under service of science, and we have to be aware of that.

The concept of"molecular allergy" is not only to request the laboratory technician for determinations of sIgE by sophisticated methods, but also to understand these techniques and apply all this knowledge to benefit our patients. The usage of allergen-based diagnostic methodologies must reach the patient and not only remain for investigation.

Acknowledgements

We thank Jesus Esteban Mendoza for the art and edition of the images included in this chapter. We also thank "Conde Valenciana Foundation" for providing its support in publishing this work.

Author details

Alberto Salazar[1,2], Henry Velázquez-Soto[2], Julio Ayala-Balboa[2] and María C. Jiménez-Martínez[1,2]*

*Address all correspondence to: mcjimenezm@bq.unam.mx

1 Department of Biochemistry, Faculty of Medicine, National Autonomous University of Mexico, Mexico City, Mexico

2 Department of Immunology and Research Unit, Institute of Ophthalmology "Conde de Valenciana," Mexico City, Mexico

References

[1] Tanno LK, Calderon MA, Smith HE, Sanchez-Borges M, Sheikh A, Demoly G, et al. Dissemination of definitions and concepts of allergic and hypersensitivity conditions. World Allergy Organ Journal. 2016;**9**(24):1-9. DOI: 10.1186/s40413-016-0115-2

[2] Fritzsching B. Personalized medicine in allergic asthma: At the crossroads of allergen immunotherapy and "Biologicals". Frontiers in Pediatrics. 2017;**5**(31):1-4. DOI: 10.3389/fped.2017.00031

[3] Salter HH. On Asthma: Ist Pathology and Treatment. 2nd ed. London: Churchill; 1868. p. 236

[4] Pirquet C. Der diagnostische wert der kutanen tuberkulinreaktion bei der tuberkulose des kindesalters auf grund von 100 sektionen. Wien klin Wshcr. 1907;**20**:1123

[5] Smith HL. Buckwheat-poisoning with report of a case in man. Archives of Internal Medicine. 1909;**3**:350

[6] Schloss OM. A case of allergy to common foods. American Journal of Diseases of Children. 1912;**3**:341

[7] Cohen SG, Frankland AW, Dworetzky M. Noon and Freeman on prophylactic inoculation against hay fever. The Journal of Allergy and Clinical Immunology. 2003;**111**(5):1142-1150

[8] Fineman AH. Studies in hypersensitiveness. XXIII: A comparative study of the intradermal, scratch and conjunctival tests in determining the degree of pollen sensitivity. Journal of Immunology. 1926;**11**(6):465-476

[9] Hansel FK. Coseasonal intracutaneous treatment of hay fever. Journal of Allergy. 1941;**12**:457

[10] Calderón-Ezquerro MC, Guerrero-Guerra C, Martínez-López B, Fuentes-Rojas F, Téllez-Unzueta F, López-Espinoza ED, et al. First airborne pollen calendar for Mexico City and its relationship with bioclimatic factors. Aerobiologia. 2016;**32**(2):225-244

[11] Rojo J, Rapp A, Lara B, Sabariego S, Fernández-González F, Pérez-Badia R. Characterisation of the airborne pollen spectrum in Guadalajara (central Spain) and estimation of the potential allergy risk. Environmental Monitoring and Assessment. 2016;**188**(3):130. DOI: 10.1007/s10661-016-5129-2

[12] Heinzerling L, Mari A, Bergmann KC, Bresciani M, Burbach G, Darsow U, et al. The skin prick test—European standards. Clinical and Translational Allergy. 2013;**3**(1):3. DOI: 10.1186/2045-7022-3-3

[13] Larenas-Linnemann D, Ortega-Martell JA, Del Río-Navarro B, Rodríguez-Pérez N, Arias-Cruz A, Estrada A, et al. Mexican clinical practice guidelines of immunotherapy 2011. Revista Alergia Mexico. 2011;**58**(1):3-75

[14] Cohen S, King JR. Skin tests: A historic trail. Immunology and Allergy Clinics of North America. 2001;**21**(2):191-249

[15] Haahtela T, Burbach GJ, Bachert C, Bindslev-Jensen C, Bonini S, Bousquet J, et al. Clinical relevance is associated with allergen-specific wheal size in skin prick testing. Clinical & Experimental Allergy. 2014;**44**(3):407-416. DOI: 10.1111/cea.12240

[16] Ishizaka K, Ishizaka T. Identification of gamma-E-antibodies as a carrier of reaginic activity. Journal of Immunology. 1967;**99**(6):1187-1198

[17] Seagroatt V, Anderson SG. The second international reference preparation for human serum immunoglobulin E and the first British standard for human serum immunoglobulin E. Journal of Biological Standardization. 1981;**9**(4):431-437

[18] Chou TY, Wu KY, Shieh CC, Wang JY. The clinical efficacy of in vitro allergen-specific IgE antibody test in the diagnosis of allergic children with asthma. Acta Paediatrica Taiwanica. 2002;**43**(1):35-39

[19] Matysiak J, Matysiak J, Bręborowicz A, Dereziński P, Kokot ZJ. The correlation between anti phospholipase A2 specific IgE and clinical symptoms after a bee sting in beekeepers. Postepy Dermatologii i Alergologii. 2016;**33**(3):206-210. DOI: 10.5114/ada.2016.60613

[20] Wainstein BK, Yee A, Jelley D, Ziegler M, Ziegler JB. Combining skin prick, immediate skin application and specific-IgE testing in the diagnosis of peanut allergy in children. Pediatric Allergy and Immunology. 2007;**18**(3):231-239

[21] Wide L, Bennich H, Johansson SG. Diagnosis of allergy by an in-vitro test for allergen antibodies. Lancet. 1967;**2**(7526):1105-1107

[22] Berg T, Bennich H, Johansson SG. In vitro diagnosis of atopic allergy. I. A comparison between provocation tests and the radioallergosorbent test. International Archives of Allergy and Immunology. 1971;**40**(6):770-778

[23] Lequin RM. EnzymeImmunoassay(EIA)/Enzyme linked immunosorbent assay (ELISA. Clinical Chemistry. 2005;**51**(12):2415-2418

[24] Johansson SG, Berglund A, Kjellman NI. Comparison of IgE values as determined by different solid phase radioimmunoassay methods. Clinical Allergy. 1976;**6**(1):91-98

[25] Bayne NK, Mathews KP. Determination of total IgE by ELISA in tubes and plates compared with PRIST. Clinical Biochemistry. 1982;**15**(3):167-169

[26] Strachan R., Wood J, Hirschmann R. Synthesis and properties of 4-Methyl -2-oxo-1,2-benzopyran-7-yl β-D-galactoside (Galactoside of 4-methylumbelliferone. Journal of Organic Chemistry. 1962;**27**:1074-1075

[27] Wood RA, Segall N, Ahlstedt S, Williams PB. Accuracy of IgE antibody laboratory results. Annals of Allergy, Asthma & Immunology. 2007;**99**(1):34-41

[28] Szecsi PB, Stender S. Comparison of immunoglobulin E measurements on IMMULITE and ImmunoCAP in samples consisting of allergen-specific mouse-human chimeric monoclonal antibodies towards allergen extracts and four recombinant allergens. International Archives of Allergy and Immunology. 2013;**162**(2):131-134. DOI: 10.1159/000353276

[29] Shyur SD, Jan RL, Webster JR, Chang P, Lu YJ, Wang JY. Determination of multiple allergen-specific IgE by microfluidic immunoassay cartridge in clinical settings. Pediatric Allergy and Immunology. 2010;**21**(4 Pt 1):623-633. DOI: 10.1111/j.1399-3038.2009.00956.x

[30] Jahn-Schmid B, Harwanegg C, Hiller R, Bohle B, Ebner C, Scheiner O, et al. Allergen microarray: Comparison of microarray using recombinant allergens with conventional diagnostic methods to detect allergen-specific serum immunoglobulin E. Clinical & Experimental Allergy. 2003;**33**(10):1443-1449

[31] Önell A, Whiteman A, Nordlund B, Baldracchini F, Mazzoleni G, Hedlin G, et al. Allergy testing in children with persistent asthma: Comparison of four diagnostic methods. Allergy. 2017;**72**(4):590-597. DOI: 10.1111/all.13047

[32] Bonini M, Marcomini L, Gramiccioni C, Tranquilli C, Melioli G, Canonica GW, et al. Microarray evaluation of specific IgE to allergen components in elite athletes. Allergy. 2012;**67**(12):1557-1564. DOI: 10.1111/all.12029

[33] Westwood M, Ramaekers B, Lang S, Armstrong N, Noake C, de Kock S, et al. ImmunoCAP® ISAC and Microtest for multiplex allergen testing in people with difficult to manage allergic disease: A systematic review and cost analysis. Health Technology Assessment. 2016;**20**(67):1-178. DOI: 10.3310/hta20670

[34] Kahlert H, Petersen A, Becker WM, Schlaak M. Epitope analysis of the allergen ovalbumin (Gal d II) with monoclonal antibodies and patients' IgE. Molecular Immunology. 1992;**29**(10):1191-1201

[35] Pahr S, Selb R, Weber M, Focke-Tejkl M, Hofer G, Dordić A, et al. Biochemical, biophysical and IgE-epitope characterization of the wheat food allergen, Tri a 37. PLoS One. 2014;**9**(11):e111483. DOI: 10.1371/journal.pone.0111483

[36] de Leon MP, Glaspole IN, Drew AC, Rolland JM, O'Hehir RE, Suphioglu C. Immunological analysis of allergenic cross-reactivity between peanut and tree nuts. Clinical & Experimental Allergy. 2003;**33**(9):1273-1280

[37] Bonds RS, Midoro-Horiuti T, Goldblum R. A structural basis for food allergy: The role of cross-reactivity. Current Opinion in Allergy and Clinical Immunology. 2008;**8**(1):82-86. DOI: 10.1097/ACI.0b013e3282f4177e

[38] García BE, Lizaso MT. Cross-reactivity syndromes in food allergy. Journal of Investigational Allergology and Clinical Immunology. 2011;**21**(3):162-170

[39] Popescu FD. Cross-reactivity between aeroallergens and food allergens. World Journal of Methodology. 2015;**5**(2):31-50. DOI: 10.5662/wjm.v5.i2.31

[40] Kuehn A, Codreanu-Morel F, Lehners-Weber C, Doyen V, Gomez-André SA, Bienvenu F, et al. Cross-reactivity to fish and chicken meat - a new clinical syndrome. Allergy. 2016;**71**(12):1772-1781. DOI: 10.1111/all.12968

[41] Herzenberg LA, Parks D, Sahaf B, Perez O, Roederer M, Herzenberg LA. The history and future of the fluorescence activated cell sorter and flow cytometry: A view from Stanford. Clinical Chemistry. 2002;**48**(10):1819-1827

[42] Cho SH, Godin JM, Chen CH, Qiao W, Lee H, Lo YH. Review article: Recent advancements in optofluidic flow cytometer. Biomicrofluidics. 2010;**4**(4):43001. DOI: 10.1063/1.3511706

[43] Herzenberg LA, Tung J, Moore WA, Herzenberg LA, Parks DR. Interpreting flow cytometry data: A guide for the perplexed. Nature Immunology. 2006;**7**(7):681-685

[44] Galicia-Carreón J, Santacruz C, Ayala-Balboa J, Robles-Contreras A, Perez-Tapia SM, Garfias Y, et al. An imbalance between frequency of CD4+CD25+FOXP3+ regulatory T cells and CCR4+ and CCR9+ circulating helper T cells is associated with active perennial allergic conjunctivitis. Clinical and Developmental Immunology. 2013;**2013**:919742. DOI: 10.1155/2013/919742

[45] Freer G, Rindi L. Intracellular cytokine detection by fluorescence-activated flow cytometry: Basic principles and recent advances. Methods. 2013;**61**(1):30-38. DOI: 10.1016/j.ymeth.2013.03.035

[46] Tang W, Smith SG, Salter B, Oliveria JP, Mitchell P, Nusca GM, et al. Allergen-induced increases in Interleukin-25 and Interleukin-25 receptor expression in mature eosinophils from atopic asthmatics. International Archives of Allergy and Immunology. 2016;**170**(4):234-242

[47] Szegedi K, Kremer AE, Kezic S, Teunissen MB, Bos JD, Luiten RM, et al. Increased frequencies of IL-31-producing T cells are found in chronic atopic dermatitis skin. Experimental Dermatology. 2012;**21**(6):431-436. DOI: 10.1111/j.1600-0625.2012.01487.x

[48] Magaña D, Aguilar G, Linares M, Ayala-Balboa J, Santacruz C, Chávez R, et al. Intracellular IL-4, IL-5, and IFN-γ as the main characteristic of CD4+CD30+ T cells after allergen stimulation in patients with vernal keratoconjunctivitis. Molecular Vision. 2015;**21**:443-450

[49] Antal-Szalmás P, Nagy B Jr, Debreceni IB, Kappelmayer J. Measurement of soluble biomarkers by flow cytometry. Electronic Journal of IFCC2013;**23**(4):1315-1342

[50] Santacruz C, Linares M, Garfias Y, Loustaunau LM, Pavon L, Perez-Tapia SM, et al. Expression of IL-8, IL-6 and IL-1β in tears as a main characteristic of the immune response in human microbial keratitis. International Journal of Molecular Sciences. 2015;**16**(3):4850-4864. DOI: 10.3390/ijms16034850

[51] Hu J, Leng X, Hu Y, Atik A, Song X, Li Z, et al. The features of inflammation factors concentrations in aqueous humor of polypoidal choroidal vasculopathy. PLoS One. 2016;**11**(1):e0147346. DOI: 10.1371/journal.pone.0147346

[52] Aktas Cetin E, Cosan F, Kucuksezer UC, Bilgic S, Cagatay Y, Gul A, et al. Behçet's disease: Immunological relevance with arthritis of ankylosing spondylitis. Rheumatology International. 2013;**33**(3):733-741. DOI: 10.1007/s00296-012-2446-9

[53] McHugh TM. Flow microsphere immunoassay for the quantitative and simultaneous detection of multiple soluble analytes. Methods in Cell Biology. 1994;**42**(Pt B):575-595

[54] Telford WG. Near infrared lasers in flow cytometry. Methods. 2015;**82**:12-20. DOI: 10.1016/j.ymeth.2015.03.010

[55] Wester K, Jönsson AK, Spigset O, Druid H, Hägg S. Incidence of fatal adverse drug reactions: A population based study. British Journal of Clinical Pharmacology. 2008;**65**(4): 573-579

[56] Elzagallaai AA, Greff MJ, Rieder MJ. Adverse drug reactions in children: The double edged sword of therapeutics. 2017;**101**:725-735. DOI: 10.1002/cpt.677

[57] Abuaf N, Rostane H, Rajoely B, Gaouar H, Autegarden JE, Leynadier F, et al. Comparison of two basophil activation markers CD63 and CD203c in the diagnosis of amoxicillin allergy. Clinical & Experimental Allergy. 2008;**38**(6):921-928. DOI: 10.1111/j.1365-2222.2008.02960.x

[58] Stain C, Stockinger H, Scharf M, Jäger U, Gössinger H, Lechner K, et al. Human blood basophils display a unique phenotype including activation linked membrane structures. Blood. 1987;**70**(6):1872-1879

[59] Bühring HJ, Streble A, Valent P. The basophil-specific ectoenzyme E-NPP3 (CD203c) as a marker for cell activation and allergy diagnosis. International Archives of Allergy and Immunology. 2004;**133**(4):317-329

[60] Boumiza R, Debard AL, Monneret G. The basophil activation test by flow cytometry: Recent developments in clinical studies, standardization and emerging perspectives. Clinical and Molecular Allergy. 2005;**3**:9

[61] Erdmann SM, Sachs B, Kwiecien R, Moll-Slodowy S, Sauer I, Merk HF. The basophil activation test in wasp venom allergy: Sensitivity, specificity and monitoring specific immunotherapy. Allergy. 2004;**59**(10):1102-1109

[62] Khan FM, Ueno-Yamanouchi A, Serushago B, Bowen T, Lyon AW, Lu C, et al. Basophil activation test compared to skin prick test and fluorescence enzyme immunoassay for aeroallergen-specific Immunoglobulin-E. Allergy, Asthma & Clinical Immunology. 2012;**8**:1. DOI: 10.1186/1710-1492-8-1

[63] Simons FE, Ebisawa M, Sanchez-Borges M, Thong BY, Worm M, Tanno LK, et al. 2015 update of the evidence base: World Allergy Organization anaphylaxis guideline. World Allergy Organ Journal. 2015;**8**:1. DOI: 10.1186/s40413-015-0080-1

[64] Smith WB, Guida L, Sun Q, Korpelainen EI, van den Heuvel C, Gillis D, et al. Neutrophils activated by granulocyte-macrophage colony-stimulating factor express receptors for interleukin-3 which mediate class II expression. Blood. 1995;**86**(10):3938-3944

Chapter 6

Current Issues on Immunotherapy in Children

Ivana Djuric-Filipovic, Snezana Zivanovic,
Gordana Kostić, Djordje Filipovic,
Marco Caminti and Zorica Zivkovic

Additional information is available at the end of the chapter

http://dx.doi.org/10.5772/intechopen.70298

Abstract

Therapy of allergic diseases in children implicates avoidance of allergens, standard pharmacotherapy, and immunotherapy. Immunotherapy is the only treatment for allergic diseases with the ability to change the natural course of the disease, thus stopping its further progression as well as the development of new allergic diseases and new sensibilizations. The objective of this chapter is to give insight into the latest data on immunotherapy in treating children with allergic diseases. Methods: The study involved a search for relevant articles on the MEDLINE and PubMed up to 2017. Results: Numerous studies have shown that the sublingual application of allergen-specific immunotherapy is adequate, safe, and efficient in the therapy of immunoglobulin E (IgE)-mediated allergic diseases of the respiratory tract in children, but there are still some questions to be solved concerning the usage of SLIT in children younger than 5 years old, SLIT for polysensitized patients, duration of SLIT, long-lasting effects of SLIT. Conclusions: In order to improve the clinical efficacy of SLIT, we are looking for new routes of administration, new allergens, new protocols as well as combination of SLIT with other immune modulatory treatments.

Keywords: allergen immunotherapy, children, asthma, allergic rhinitis

1. Introduction

1.1. Epidemiology of asthma and rhinitis

With a global prevalence of 6.9% (ranging from 3.8 in Asia-Pacific and Northern and Eastern Europe to 11.3% in North America), asthma is one of the most common chronic diseases in children, adolescent, and adults [1]. The prevalence rate of allergic rhinitis, asthma, and eczema in Serbia has been investigated as a part of the International Study of Asthma and Allergies Phase Three. The study included around 14,000 from 5 regional centers different geographical and urban characteristics (children both from urban and rural areas participated). Investigators analyzed the prevalence of allergic diseases in two age groups (the first one preschool children aged 6–7 years old and the second one children between the age of 13–14 years old. The prevalence of asthma was 6.59% in younger age group, whereas the prevalence in older age group was around 5.36%. Note that 7.17% of preschool children and 14.89% of school children were diagnosed allergic rhinitis. Overall, asthma prevalence was 5.91%, rhinitis 11.46%, and eczema 14.27% [2]. The growing worldwide burden of allergic diseases is properly defined as the "allergy epidemic." The German epidemiological Multicenter Allergy Study (MAS) suggested an age-related evolution of atopic and allergic diseases, usually named "atopic march." In fact, on epidemiological bases, infantile eczema and food allergy usually precede the onset of allergic airway disease (rhinitis and asthma). It is also interesting to point out that unlike other common chronic diseases such as diabetes mellitus or hypertension, it is well established that the development of allergic diseases start just after birth or according to some authors maybe earlier in prenatal period [3]. The incidence of asthma is the highest in preschool and early school age with an improvement in symptoms and a decrease in prevalence afterwards, but with one more pic in incidence in adolescents' period especially in female teenagers mainly due to hormone disturbance. It is well known that allergic diseases are multi factorial which means that in their pathophysiology both genetic and environmental factors are included. Atopic family history is one of the most important risk factors for the development of asthma. MAS cohort study analyzed the main risk factors for persistent asthma/wheeze in an early adolescent's period. According to the results from this huge study wheezing before the age of 3 as well as wheezing after the age of 6, accompanied with early atopic dermatitis, positive family history of atopic diseases and positive allergy tests, particular to perennial allergens represent the main risk factors [4, 5].

Although according to birth cohort studies data we are aware that genetic burden has an important influence in allergies development and despite lots of efforts, we have still failed to identify responsible genes. Many factors in the environment contribute to the development of allergies (e.g., diet, immunizations, antibiotics, pets, and tobacco smoke), but we do not know how to modify the environment to reduce the risks [6]. According to several epidemiological studies, a decline in microbial diversity was proposed to have an important role in allergic epidemic, best summarized in hygiene hypothesis, and nowadays defined as "biodiversity hypothesis." Identification of prenatal and early postnatal risk factors is of a great importance for early prevention and successful intervention. Two recent studies showed that reduce food diversity in early childhood can be associated with atopic sensitization and allergic diseases later on. It is also suggested that high "antigen burden" in early life can be a protective factor necessary to "educate" the immune system and to prevent childhood allergic diseases. Early allergy prevention that includes: administrations of probiotics to pregnant mothers and to high-risk children, oral or intranasal extracts, and earlier introduction of foods is still matter of a debate due to conflicting results [7, 8]. Despite many different options are currently available for the diagnostic workup and management, the burden of allergic airway diseases still represents a major health problem in childhood. It is a very well known that allergic diseases are multifactorial in terms that both genetic and environmental and risk factors are involved in its pathogenesis. Taking about different endo- or phenotype is very common when we analyze these diseases. Looking for a better quality of life (QOL) and disease of overall morbidity and mortality rate seek further investigation on every single individual risk factor that can have even the smallest impact on the disease development. Searching for a new and more individualized treatment for allergic diseases most of current research is focusing on the identification of biological and clinical predictive markers of allergy and asthma onset [9].

2. Diagnostic tools and monitoring

Despite many different diagnostic tools for allergic disease it still remains a challenge especially in infants and toddlers. Skin tests represent an important diagnostic tool in workup of many allergic diseases. These tests are mainly used for the diagnosis of inhalant allergies, but nowadays there are more and more tendencies to use this kind of tests for allergies to food, venom, occupational agents, and drugs. Skin prick tests (SPTs) and intradermal tests still represent the cornerstone of the diagnosis of IgE-mediated (type I) allergies. They are easy to perform, cheap and allow a fast reading, usually performed in outpatient clinics. Performing skin prick tests needs a specific training, especially for intradermal and epicutaneous tests with nonstandard allergens, that are not usually performed in children population. Special precautions that have to be considered before performing skin prick tests include the usage of some drugs, skin conditions and in adolescents and adults pregnancy. Before performing *in vivo* skin prick tests patients are not allowed to take drugs such as antihistamines at least several days because it is well known that these kinds of drugs could mask positive results of type I reactions, on the other side conditions like pressure urticaria or dermographism are able to provoke false positive results. For that reason using positive control histamine and negative control saline solution are crucial for results interpretations. Skin prick tests (SPT) are one of the most important diagnostic tools in asthma and AR diagnosis with sensitization to inhalant allergens. They can get prompt information on sensitization to inhalant allergens such as pollen, house dust mites, pets, to a lesser extent molds. Recommendation for SPTs is available with more or less variation in many climate and geographical areas. As they are very cheap and easy to perform SPTs are of a great importance especially in undeveloped or developing countries. Here, it is also interesting to mention that in tropical areas standard SPTs battery should include typical tropical allergens such as Blomia tropical. In southeastern and Western Europe standard allergens for preforming SPTs usually include following allergen solutions: tree, ragweed, and grass pollen, house dust mite, molds, cockroach, dogs, and cats dander. Before starting allergen-specific immunotherapy SPTs have to be performed [10–14]. Nasal and bronchial provocation test are indicated for patients with typical clinical symptoms and signs of allergic rhinitis and/ or asthma but with negative *in vivo* skin prick tests [15]. Those tests should be performed exclusively by a well-trained staff at the allergy departments. They are very important for distinguishing allergic and nonallergic rhinitis as well as for the diagnosis of local allergic rhinitis (LAR)—typical clinical history of allergic rhinitis with positive nasal provocation test, usually with elevated eosinophils in nasal smear, but with negative skin prick or/and *in vitro* allergy tests [16]. *In vitro* allergy tests are cornerstone of allergy diagnostic especially in the pediatric population. All children with positive clinical history of allergic diseases (atopic dermatitis, allergic rhinitis, and/or asthma) should be evaluated, particularly those with positive uni- or bilateral family history of atopic diseases. Determinations of total IgE, followed with evaluation of the allergen-specific antibody levels are precede the introduction of allergen-specific immunotherapy. It is also a very important to be mentioned that the interpretation of the allergy tests should be strictly done in the light of clinical history of a certain patients. Novel diagnostic tools are also capable to determine sensitization to a specific pure or recombinant allergens that is of a great importance for individualized treatment approach. Sometimes this kind of tests are the most relevant to confirm the diagnosis of allergy sensitization. To data, the most commonly used system to determine allergen-specific IgE is the ImmunoCAP system that are considered as a goal standard for *in vitro* diagnosis of allergen condition. Despite great technological improvements in *in vitro* diagnostics of allergies, several problems still remain. Although elevated IgE is a marker of IgE-mediated allergy, this is not sufficient for the induction of symptoms. According to the data, more than 20% of patients with elevated IgE are in fact asymptomatic. Elevated serum IgE level is irrelevant as long as it does not bind to Fcέ receptors on effectors cells (mastocytes, eosinophils, and basophils). Positive allergen-specific IgE in serum is not sufficient to confirm allergy in all cases [17–19]. At the current state of art it is a very important to be a little bit septic about allergy diagnostic test results only based on determination of allergen-specific serum IgE levels and to consider clinical history, accompanied by adequate skin prick tests or provocation tests, which drive the diagnosis before considering allergen-specific immunotherapy inclusion. During the last decades, there has been a huge improvement in *in vitro* allergy diagnosis due to novel approaches that include molecular components. It has been already mentioned that allergen-specific tests are not enough sensitive and specific for allergy diagnosis, through the advent of molecular technology, some weaknesses, and shortcomings of classical approach that used only natural extracts could be solved. Component resolved diagnosis (CRD) of the specific IgE response provides more individual approach in diagnosis of allergic patients and better selection of patients for allergen-specific immunotherapy. It is also of a great value for monitoring of the efficacy, immunogenicity and safety of allergen-specific immunotherapy [20, 21]. Cellular allergy testing represents one more *in vitro* allergy diagnostic tool. It expands the tools of allergist to diagnose and monitor allergic diseases. The basophil activation test (BAT) is the most common used cellular allergy tests in routine clinical practice and in research. That test is able to document type I sensitization to a specific allergen, as fraction of blood basophils activated by soluble allergen. Basophil sensitivity can be used for identification the main sensitizer among cross-reacting allergens or allergen preparation as well as for monitoring progress of allergen-specific immunotherapy and anti-IgE therapy [22–24].

3. Biomarkers and prediction

Determination of a certain biomarkers that are known to be important in pathophysiology of allergic diseases can be a very useful in primary prevention, early intervention and disease course modification [25]. Currently reliable tools that can adequately predict which children will develop asthma are still lacking [26]. Nowadays identification and determination of biomarkers in diagnosis of allergic diseases represent an important step toward better understanding of a great number of different endotypes. Biomarkers are also very important for increasing drug effectiveness through a more individualized therapeutic approach. Discovering novel biomarkers or combining them with the existing one and better understanding of different asthma endo- and phenotypes are important goals in allergy research improving both allergy diagnosis and treatment [27–29]. Fractional exhaled nitric oxide FeNO is considered a very good biomarker of eosinophilic inflammation of lower airways. Many data showed that FeNO is a reliable predictor of corticosteroids responsiveness [30]. The results form the most recent studies indicated that allergen-specific immunotherapy has also an impact on the decrease of eosinophilic airway inflammation [31]. Periostin is a downstream molecule of interleukin (IL)-4 and/or IL-13 has been recently marked as a surrogate biomarker of type 2 inflammation and tissue remodeling in bronchial asthma. It has been shown that serum periostin can predict the efficacy of anti-IL-13 antibody (lebrikizumab) and anti-IgE antibody (omalizumab). Sputum eosinophils are useful for estimating the efficacy of anti-IL-5 antibody (mepolizumab) [32, 33].

4. Therapy of allergic airway disease in childhood

Although there are numerous studies, management of allergic disease is still a matter of a debate. According to the data management of allergic diseases, consider avoidance of the risk factors, treatment, and induction of tolerance. In that light the management of allergic diseases depends on how easy is to avoid the triggers, whether there are multiple triggers and how easy is to induce tolerance. The possibility to avoid certain allergen mainly depends on the nature of that allergen. For ubiquitous allergens such as house dust mites or pollens it is usually impossible to avoid, unlike for animal dander [34]. There are also some studies suggest that food allergen avoidance in pregnancy, lactation, and infancy have preventive role in the development of food allergy, and possibly other allergic diseases. The only current recommendations to prevent allergic disease are exclusive breastfeeding at least 4–6 months and if breastfeeding is insufficient or not possible, hypoallergenic formula for the high-risk infants [35–37]. The most common approach used in allergic diseases treatment is symptomatic therapy in step management strategies. Pharmacologic therapy is tailored to the primary symptom or symptoms and to the severity of symptoms without modifies the long-term outcome of allergy. The optimal utilization of pharmacologic therapies varies among regions and countries and varying preference of therapies in different populations [38, 39]. According to the clinical data, more targeted therapies include monoclonal antibodies against IgE and against various proallergic cytokines (e.g., anti-IL-5, anti-IL-13, and anti-IgE). Although expensive, these therapies are useful in the management of selected patients who are usually unresponsiveness to standard pharmacological treatment [40].

5. History of sublingual allergen-specific immunotherapy

Although all story of immunotherapy seems to be a new one, the first routes of immunotherapy dates back to 1911 when two English researchers used water solution of hay fever pollen extracts for treating hypersensitized patients. They noticed that hypodermal inoculation of specific allergen could have some benefit. Without a sound knowledge of basic and clinical immunology immunotherapy was pure empiric, not so widely used treatment for decades [41, 42]. The second very important step in the history of sublingual immunotherapy was the findings of a group of German researchers who showed that sublingual route of allergen-specific immunotherapy could be equally clinical effective as subcutaneous route [4, 43]. They performed a small double-blind placebo control crossover trail. The maximum subcutaneous tolerated dose of a house dust mite (HDM) extract was given sublingual as drops three times daily [44]. They showed an improvement in symptoms and improvement in nasal inspiratory peak flow. A few years later Scadding's and Brostoff proved a clinical efficacy of low dose sublingual immunotherapy in patients with allergic rhinitis sensitized to house dust mites in a double-blind placebo-controlled trial (DB-PCT) [45] whereas Italian allergist were the first one who showed clinical efficacy of SLIT for patients with allergic rhinitis and/or asthma sensitized also to house dust mites. Those study included both adults and children population [46]. In early 1990s, the first commercial available sublingual immune drops were developed. Since the introduction of sublingual immune drops, the scientific community has been seeking for improvement. When evaluating the findings from clinical trials with sublingual immunotherapy drops, it became clear that this therapy was more likely to be effective when administered once daily and higher doses. Moreover, pharmacokinetic studies of SLIT showed that only a very small proportion of liquid extracts was taken up into superficial layer of sublingual mucosa. Searching for a way to augment local allergen uptake sublingual rapidly dissolving tablets were developed. These tablets facilitated the delivery of high concentration of allergen in a small volume. This concept led to the clinical and commercial development of high-dose sublingual AIT using fast-dissolving tablets [47]. Early papers with sublingual allergen immunotherapy demonstrated positive results, and in 1993, the European Academy of Allergy and Clinical Immunology was the first official organization to recognize that sublingual administration could be a "promising route" for allergic desensitization. Two studies from 1999 to 2001 showed a satisfied safety profile of sublingual route for both children and adults [48–51]. From 1998, the World Health Organization recommended SLIT as an "a viable alternative to the injection route in adults" [52]. Wilson Cochrane review from 2003 analyzed 49 randomized control trials (RCTs) with 4589 children and adults affected by allergic rhinitis (with or without asthma or conjunctivitis) and proved clinical efficacy of SLIT over placebo [53]. To date, over 70 double-blind, placebo-controlled trails and several meta-analyses of sublingual allergy immunotherapy drops have been reported. It is important to note that many trails with SLIT drops or tablets were small and/or had an open label design. Over the last 10 years, however, several adequately designed and powered trails have been conducted with grass pollen, as well as with Dermatophagoides pteronyssinus (DP) in both adults and children, and have demonstrated efficacy and safety with this therapeutic approach [10, 54].

6. Clinical efficacy of SLIT still matter of a debate

Although a great number of various meta-analyses and DB-PC-RCTs have showed clinical efficacy of SLIT in children population diagnosed allergic rhinitis and/or asthma [55], due to significant clinical and methodological heterogeneity, some issues are still a matter of debate. One of the main issues to be solved is long-term efficacy, particularly after cessation of the treatment. Results from several European clinical trials in pediatric and adult patients with grass pollen-induced rhinoconjunctivitis have shown that grass AIT reduces daily rhinoconjunctivitis symptom scores compared with patients receiving only symptomatic medications. The proportion of days with minimal or no symptoms increase in patients on SLIT. The same study also showed the improvement of quality of life in children on SLIT. The beneficial effects were observed for three consecutive years of treatment as well as during the first year following cessation period, indicating a disease modifying effect and persistence of efficacy despite discontinuation of therapy [56–60]. Due to the fact that majority of atopic patients are poly sensitized, one of the most important issues to be answered is SLIT efficacy in those patients. Recent study confirmed clinical efficacy of SLIT in reducing nasal and ocular symptoms and the use of rescue medications, also observed no differences in clinical efficacy in mono- and poly-sensitized patients [61]. However, the cross-protection against unrelated allergens seems to be limited [62]. Although it passed more than a decade of proven clinical efficacy of SLIT, data of long-lasting effects are still missing. Results from a 15-year-long prospective study by Marogna et al. [63] show that long-lasting effects of SLIT are in direct correlation with the treatment's duration. Some study suggested that 4 years of SLIT may be associated with more favorable effects than 3 years of treatment [64]. As the only immune modulatory treatment for allergic diseases, preventive role of AIT is of a great interest. Some authors are very doubtful concerning the adherence and tolerability of the treatment particularly in the pediatric population [65], whereas the other one claimed that even 1 or 2 years of treatment is sufficient to mediate immunological response [66, 67]. The second important issue on SLIT is long-lasting effects. After a 12 years of follow-up period Eng et al. showed preventive effects of SLIT 6 years after the treatment termination comparing with the standard pharmacotherapy [68]. Although the best candidates for allergen-specific immunotherapy are mono sensitized patients Malling et al. in their study showed that desensibilization with the predominant allergen in polysensitized participants can be similar effective [69]. In the light of preventive effects of immunotherapy and possibility to have impact on further evolution of allergic diseases (atopic march), the opportunity to use this kind of treatment in very young children is of a great importance, but several issues have to be answered [70–72]. Immunotherapy can overcome problems related to the long-term pharmacotherapy [73], adherence and compliance to the standard treatment. Low-adherence and bad compliance to a long-term pharmacotherapy, both drug (problems with the usage of inhaled drugs) and non/drug-related factors can be overcome with the introduction of immunotherapy. All chronic diseases have an impact on quality of life due to high score of school absenteeism, impaired school performance, frequent emergency unit visits. Children with allergic diseases especially those with asthma showed low physical activity performance [74, 75]. High level of anxiety as well as higher incidence of depression and other physiological disorders can be seen in children and adolescents with asthma, allergic rhinitis and atopic dermatitis. A certain number of studies confirmed the impact of SLIT on all previous mentioned aspects of quality of life [76, 77].

7. Safety and tolerability of SLIT in allergic children

Over the last 20 years, sublingual allergen immunotherapy has gained popularity based on controlled trails that have demonstrated a favorable safety profile [78, 79]. Although a great number of DB-PC-RCT showed clinical efficacy of SCIT since the British Committee on Safety of Medicines in the UK reported 26 SCIT-related anaphylactic deaths between 1957 and 1986, the interest for alternative routes constantly grows. The risk of subcutaneous immunotherapy (SCIT)-related systemic adverse events (SAEs) still represent a major concern that may, sometimes limit the use of this effective treatment, especially in the pediatric population. On the other side the overall safety of SLIT has been widely proven and accepted [80]. Moreover, Nichani study showed that SLIT can be safely administered to patients who previously experienced systemic reactions in response to subcutaneous allergen immunotherapy.

According to double-blind placebo-controlled-randomized clinical trials (DB-PC-RCTs) for allergic asthma, allergic rhinitis or allergic rhinoconjunctivitis [80–84] and real-life studies only several life-threatening and nonlife-threatening severe systemic reaction related to SLIT are reported [50, 85–87]. Overall prevalence of systemic adverse events was lower than 20% in DB-PC-RCT, whereas the prevalence of severe systemic reactions was between 1 and 2% of total recorded events [88–93]. Most commonly postmarketing surveys reported mild to moderate usually self-resolved systemic reactions [94, 95]. A very important issue concerning SLIT particularly in the pediatric population is to define risk factors for developing systemic reactions. Up to now several potential risk factors are defined: inadequate administration conditions (use of non-standardized extracts, administration of products containing a mixture of many allergens, overdosing [92]), and/or patient-related nonspecific risk factors (include cardiovascular diseases and long-term therapy with noncardioselective beta-blockers) that are very uncommon in children [96]. Those conditions are considered as special precaution, but not contraindication for SLIT introduction. On the other side uncontrolled asthma or severe asthma, oral lesion, or acute infections can represent temporary contraindication for SLIT. Although previous systemic reaction due to SCIT were considered as absolute contraindication for all kinds of immunotherapy, results from recent studies showed that they do not represent risk factors for further usage of other kinds of ASIT including sublingual [96]. Local adverse reactions are most common SLIT-related side effects although it is not very easy to record them as it is not usually including in postmarketing analysis nor in DB-PC-RCT [50, 85–88]. Its prevalence varies from 50 to 80% and they include oropharyngeal and gastro-intestinal reactions such as itching, pruritus, and eczema in oral mucosa and/or diarrhoea, vomitus, and abdominal pain [97–99].

The second issue that is also of a great importance is a matter of tolerability that can have a great impact on overall clinical outcomes [100]. Both systemic and local adverse events may have influence on treatment discontinuation as they are most common after the first administration. In order to improve adherence clinicians should be well educated and trained to recognize local and systemic adverse events and to give also patients adequate explanation how to deal with them, although SLIT has much better safety profile compared with subcutaneous allergen-specific immunotherapy. WAO proposal on grading local adverse events can help to achieve better tolerance and adherence [96].

8. Quality of life studies

According to many DB-PC-RCT, real-life studies and meta-analysis quality of life (QOL) is a very important issue for children and adults with allergic diseases. As it has been already mentioned, their quality of life is not so often satisfied particularly in school-aged period [101]. Standard pharmacotherapy treats only symptoms but not the disease itself, nor the quality of life. Although lots of studies proved clinical efficacy of SLIT, only a small part of them take QOL in consideration. One of them is Ciprandi et al. study [102] that has showed the improvement of QOL in polysensitized patients with AR and/or asthma treated with SLIT. Bousquet et al. study of DB-PC-RCT proved that patients on SLIT had a better QOL compared with the group of patients on placebo [103]. However, the results from the studies are controversial. While Bousquet et al. and Ciprandi et al. showed the improvement of the QOL in SLIT groups, Khinchi et al. found no statistical significant difference in QOL scores among three groups, that is, SLIT, SCIT, and placebo, using a 36-item short-form health survey (SF-36) questionnaire [104].

9. Oral tolerance

The mechanism of action of the allergen-specific immunotherapy is very complicated and still remained unexplained. For an easier understanding of the mechanism of action of ASIT, we divided the immune response to early and late immunological response. In the early phase of immunotherapy (induction phase) there is a decrease in the number of tissue mast cells, eosinophils and basophils followed by a decrease in the release of their cell mediators [105]. Reduction of the number of basophils induced by the oral regulation of the H2 receptor leads to the inhibition of FcεRI-mediated histamine suppression and other mediators. In the first phase of the immune response, the synthesis of IgG4 and IgA is increased [106]. IgG4 blocks the interaction of IgE and allergens as well as the presentation of allergen to T cells. In the late phase, after one to several months, the immune response from Th2 to Th1 is reoriented, as well as the increase in the number and function of both types of T-regulatory cells (T-reg): natural (nT-reg) and inducible (iT-reg) [107]. iT-reg originated from naive $CD4^+$ T lymphocytes and they are the most important source of IL-10, which is an important factor in peripheral tolerance [108, 109], because it inhibits IgE production from one, and on the other hand stimulates IgG4 secretion and in this way directly inhibits the activity of allergen-specific T lymphocytes [110]. The nT-reg cells ($CD4^+$, $CD25^+$ and $FOXP3^+$ (Forkhead box protein 3)) are thymus origin and exhibit synergistic effects with iT-reg cells [111] exposing high levels of IL-10 and TGF-beta [112]. T-reg stimulates the proliferation and differentiation of IL-10-secreting dendritic cells, which have a crucial role in the activation and differentiation of different subtypes of T cells. Reducing the number of cell mastocytes, eosinophils, and basophils, increasing IgG4 and IgA synthesis, re-orientation from Th2 to Th1, increasing the number, and function of IL-10 producing T-reg cells play a significant role in the development of immune tolerance and long-lasting immunotherapy effect on the overall immune function and on the immune response to allergens [113–116].

10. Future perspectives

As it mentioned above clinical efficacy of immunotherapy has been proven in a great number of clinical studies but there are still some issues to be discussed. Recent studies are more focused on the usage of recombinant allergen-based immunotherapy that will possible makes allergy vaccines more safe, convenient, and effective. Recombinant-allergen vaccines also contain defined amounts of the allergen components, and the composition can be tailored according to patient's sensitizations. Both recombinant allergen-diagnostic tests and immunotherapy lead to more personalized and stratified treatment of different allergic entities. Recombinant allergen-based vaccines have been developed and successfully evaluated for several respiratory allergen sources including food allergies [117–120]. The second approach for minimizing side effects and improves compliance is the usage of peptide immunotherapy that has been proven in many studies as effective in treating patients with different respiratory allergies [121]. Data from the studies showed that this kind of immunotherapy is clinical effective for months to years after a short course of treatment. Some studies also investigate new routes of administration such as intralymphatic and epicutaneous. Although it is proven as safe and efficacy, both routes require further clinical investigation [122, 123]. Recently, scientists have exploited the immune system to produce antibodies from single B cell clones, heralding the era of monoclonal antibodies. Biological agents (biologicals or biologics) bring revolution in the treatment of many rheumatic and immunological disorders and are currently being assessed for allergic disorders. Better understanding the endotypes and phenotypes of allergic disease may lead to specifically targeting the responsible molecular mechanism by a biological. The mechanism of biologicals implies the inhibition of a specific molecule involved in allergic inflammation, without weakening immunity against viruses and bacteria. The design and use of biologicals requires a profound understanding of the mechanisms underlying allergy. Several biologicals are being assessed in clinical trials, including biologicals inhibiting interleukin (IL)-4, IL-5, IL-9, IL-13, and immunoglobulin E, but most of them are still being tested in clinical trials, involving patients with allergic asthma, allergic rhinitis, food allergy, urticaria, atopic eczema, and diseases with high eosinophil counts. It is to be expected that biologicals will replace or reduce the use of the currently prescribed unspecific pharmacotherapy of allergic inflammation. Better understanding of disease endotypes, identification of novel biomarkers, and discovery of novel biologicals are the cornerstones of the modern approach in treating allergic diseases [124–127].

11. Conclusion

According to a great number of clinical studies, allergen-specific immunotherapy in combination with asthma and anti-allergic medication is clinically effective in treating children with respiratory allergies. Respecting the newest data, SLIT can be used not only in children with stable asthma, but also in those with uncontrolled asthma but then in combination with anti-IgE-omalizubam treatment. AIT in children can even bring more benefits. At first, data suggested that SLIT reduced the usage of corticosteroids that can have deep negative impact on child development. The second benefit is the possibility of AIT to change the natural course of allergic diseases in terms of asthma prevention in children with allergic rhinitis. The problem of SLIT, especially in the young population of children and adolescents, is compliance that can be possibly overcome with the introduction of ultra-rush and rush protocols. Investigating the various effects of immunotherapy based on the developmental stage of children and adolescents can help to identify the optimal dose, frequency, treatment duration, and age for starting to treatment. Better selection of well responders based on endotype-driven approach is expected to increase both efficacy and safety.

Acknowledgements

A major portion of the chapter borrows from authors' previous publications [9, 54, 77] (with the permission of all the authors).

Funding

This study was supported by the Ministry of Education, Science and Technological Development of the Republic of Serbia, Grant No. III41004 and by COST ACTION BM1407.

Author details

Ivana Djuric-Filipovic[1]*, Snezana Zivanovic[2], Gordana Kostić[3], Djordje Filipovic[4], Marco Caminti[5] and Zorica Zivkovic[6,7]

*Address all correspondence to: drivanica@yahoo.com

1 Sanofi Pasteur, Vaccine Division of Sanofi Aventis Group, Belgrade, Serbia

2 Faculty of Medicine, University of Nis, Pediatric Internal Diseases Clinic, Clinical Center of Nis, Niš

3 Faculty of Medical Science, University of Kragujevac, Children's Hospital-Clinical Centre Kragujevac, Kragujevac, Serbia

4 Institute for Emergency Medical Care, Belgrade, Serbia

5 Allergy Unit Asthma Center, Verona University Hospital, Verona, Italy

6 Children's Hospital for Lung Diseases and Tuberculosis, Medical Center "Dr Dragiša Mišović," Belgrade, Serbia

7 Faculty of Pharmacy, University Business Academy in Novi Sad, Novi Sad, Serbia

References

[1] Lai CK, Beasley R, Crane J, Foliaki S, Shah J, Weiland S. International study of asthma and allergies in childhood phase three study group. Global variation in the prevalence and severity of asthmasymptoms: Phase three of the International Study of Asthma and Allergies in Childhood (ISAAC). Thorax. 2009;**64**:476-483. DOI: 10.1136/thx.2008.106609. [PMID: 19237391]

[2] Zivkovic Z, Vukasinovic Z, Cerovic S, Radulovic S, Zivanovic S, Panic E, et al. Prevalence of childhood asthma and allergies in Serbia and Montenegro. World Journal of Pediatrics. 2010;**6**(4):331-336. DOI: 10.1007/s12519-010-0207-y. [PMID: 20549414]

[3] Gough H, Grabenhenrich L, Reich A, et al. Allergic multimorbidity of asthma, rhinitis and eczema over 20 years in the German birth cohort MAS. Pediatric Allergy and Immunology. 2015;**26**:431-437

[4] Grabenhenrich LB, Gough H, Reich A, Eckers N, Zepp F, Nitsche O, et al. Early-life determinants of asthma from birth to age 20 years: A German birth cohort study. The Journal of Allergy and Clinical Immunology. 2014;**33**:979-988

[5] Hatzler L, Penetta V, Lau S, Wagner P, Bergmann RL, Illi S, et al. Molecular spreading and predictive value of preclinical IgE response to Phleum pretense in children with hay fever. The Journal of Allergy and Clinical Immunology. 2012;**130**:894-901

[6] Holguin F. The atopic march: IgE is not the only road. The Lancet Respiratory Medicine. 2014;**2**:88-90

[7] Matricardi PM. 99th Dahlem conference on infection, inflammation and chronic inflammatory disorders: Controversial aspects of the 'hygiene hypothesis'. Clinical & Experimental Immunology. 2010;**160**:98-105

[8] Haahtela T, Holgate S, Pawankar R, et al. The biodiversity hypothesis and allergic disease. WAO position paper. World Allergy Organization Journal. 2013;**6**:3

[9] Caminati M, Duric-Filipovic I, Arasi S, Peroni DG, Zivkovic Z, Senna G. Respiratory allergies in childhood: Recent advances and future challenges. Pediatric Allergy and Immunology. 2015;**26**:702-710. M21

[10] Živković Z, Cerović S, Djurić-Filipović I, Vukašinović Z, Jocić-Stojanović J, Bajec-Opančina A. Clinical implications and facts about allergic rhinitis (AR) in children. In: Kowalski M, editor. Allergic Rhinitis. InTech; 2012. ISBN: 978-953-51-0288-5. Available from: http://www.intechopen.com/books/allergic-rhinitis/allergic-rhinitis-in-childhood-clinical-implications-and-allergen-specific-immunotherapy

[11] de Monchy JG, Demoly P, Akdis CA, Cardona V, Papadopoulos NG, Schmid-Grendelmeier P, et al. Allergology in Europe, the blueprint. Allergy. 2013;**68**:1211-1218

[12] Sicherer SH, Sampson HA. Food allergy: Epidemiology, pathogenesis, diagnosis, and treatment. The Journal of Allergy and Clinical Immunology. 2014;**133**:291-307

[13] Ballmer-Weber BK. Value of allergy tests for the diagnosis of food allergy. Journal of Digestive Diseases. 2014;**32**:84-88

[14] Strohmeier B, Aberer W, Bokanovic D, Komericki P, Sturm GJ. Simultaneous intradermal testing with hymenoptera venoms is safe and more efficient than sequential testing. Allergy. 2013;**68**:542-544

[15] Diamant Z, Gauvreau GM, Cockcroft DW, Boulet LP, Sterk PJ, de Jongh FH, et al. Inhaled allergen bronchoprovocation tests. The Journal of Allergy and Clinical Immunology. 2013;**132**:1045-1055 e6

[16] Rondon C, Campo P, Togias A, Fokkens WJ, Durham SR, Powe DG, et al. Local allergic rhinitis: Concept, pathophysiology, and management. The Journal of Allergy and Clinical Immunology. 2012;**129**:1460-1467

[17] Shreffler WG. Microarrayed recombinant allergens for diagnostic testing. The Journal of Allergy and Clinical Immunology. 2011;**127**:843-849

[18] Bousquet J, Anto J, Bachert C, Bousquet PJ, Colombo P, Crameri R, et al. Factors responsible for differences between asymptomatic subjects and patients presenting and IgE sensitization to allergens: A GA-2LEN project. Allergy. 2006;**61**:671-680

[19] Crameri R. The crux with a reliable in vitro and in vivo diagnosis of allergy. Allergy. 2013;**68**:393-394

[20] Mari A. When does a protein become an allergen? Searching for a dynamic definition based on most advanced technology tools. Clinical & Experimental Allergy. 2008; **38**:1089-1094

[21] Scala E, Alessandri C, Bernardi ML, Ferrara R, Palazzo P, Pomponi D, et al. Cross-sectional survey on immunoglobulin E reactivity in 23 077 subjects using an allergenic molecule-based microarray detection system. Clinical & Experimental Allergy. 2010;**40**:911-921

[22] Hausmann OV, Gentinetta T, Bridts CH, Ebo DG. The basophil activation test in immediate-type drug allergy. Immunology and Allergy Clinics of North America. 2009;**29**:555-566

[23] Hoffmann HJ, Frandsen PM, Christensen LH, Schiøtz PO, Dahl R. Cultured human mast cells are heterogeneous for expression of the high-affinity IgE receptor FcεRI. International Archives of Allergy and Immunology. 2012;**157**:246-250

[24] Porebski G, Gschwend-Zawodniak A, Pichler WJ. In vitro diagnosis of T cell-mediated drug allergy. Clinical & Experimental Allergy. 2011;**41**:461-470

[25] Carraro S, Scheltema N, Bont L, Baraldi E. Early-life origins of chronic respiratory diseases: Understanding and promoting healthy ageing. The European Respiratory Journal. 2014;**44**:1682-1696

[26] Bannier MA, van de Kant KD, Jöbsis Q, Dompeling E. Biomarkers to predict asthma in wheezing preschool children. Clinical & Experimental Allergy. 2015;**45**:1040-1050

[27] Vijverberg SJ, Koenderman L, Koster ES, van der Ent CK, Raaijmakers JA, Maitland-van der Zee AH. Biomarkers of therapy responsiveness in asthma: Pitfalls and promises. Clinical & Experimental Allergy. 2011;**41**:615-629

[28] Szefler SJ, Wenzel S, Brown R, Erzurum SC, Fahy JV, Hamilton RG, et al. Asthma outcomes: Biomarkers. The Journal of Allergy and Clinical Immunology. 2012;**129**:S9-S23

[29] Lötvall J, Akdis CA, Bacharier LB, Bjermer L, Casale TB, Custovic A, et al. Asthma endotypes: A new approach to classification of disease entities within the asthma syndrome. The Journal of Allergy and Clinical Immunology. 2011;**127**:355-360

[30] Barnes PJ, Dweik RA, Gelb AF, Gibson PG, George SC, Grasemann H, et al. Exhaled nitric oxide in pulmonary diseases: A comprehensive review. Chest. 2010;**138**:682-692

[31] Đurić-Filipović I, Caminati M, Salvottini C, Filipović Đ, Živković Z. Effects of specific allergen immunotherapy on biological markers and clinical parameters in asthmatic children: A controlled-real life study. Clinical and Molecular Allergy. 2017;**15**:1-7 (M23)

[32] Hanania NA, Wenzel S, Rosen K, Hsieh HJ, Mosesova S, Choy DF. Exploring the effects of omalizumab in allergic asthma: An analysis of biomarkers in the EXTRA study. American Journal of Respiratory and Critical Care Medicine. 2013;**187**:804-811

[33] Kanemitsu Y, Matsumoto H, Izuhara K, Tohda Y, Kita H, Horiguchi T, et al. Increased periostin associates with greater airflow limitation in patients receiving inhaled corticosteroids. The Journal of Allergy and Clinical Immunology. 2013;**132**:305-312

[34] Rijssenbeek-Nouwens LH, Fieten KB, Bron AO, Hashimoto S, Bel EH, Weersink EJ. High-altitude treatment in atopic and nonatopic patients with severe asthma. European Respiratory Society. 2012;**40**:1374-1380

[35] Roduit C, Frei R, Depner M, Schaub B, Loss G, Genuneit J, et al. Increased food diversity in the first year of life is inversely associated with allergic diseases. The Journal of Allergy and Clinical Immunology. 2014;**133**:1056-1064

[36] Metcalfe J, Prescott SL, Palmer DJ. Randomized controlled trials investigating the role of allergen exposure in food allergy: Where are we now? Current Opinion in Allergy and Clinical Immunology. 2013;**13**:296-305

[37] Infant Feeding Advice. Australiasian Society of Allergy and Immunology [Internet]. 2008. Available from: http://www.allergy.org au/images/stories/pospapers/ascia_infantfeedingadvice_oct08.pdf

[38] Bousquet J, Khaltaev N, Cruz AA, Denburg J, Fokkens WJ, Togias A, et al. Allergic rhinitis and its impact on asthma (ARIA) 2008 update (in collaboration with the World Health Organization, GA2LEN and Aller- Gen). Allergy. 2008;**63**:S8-S160

[39] Global Initiative for Asthma (GINA). Global Strategy for Asthma Management and Prevention [Internet]. 2012. Available from: http://www.ginasthma.org/

[40] Canonica GW, Senna G, Mitchell PD, O'Byrne PM, Passalacqua G, Varricchi G. Therapeutic interventions in severe asthma. World Allergy Organization Journal. 2016;**9**(1):40

[41] Noon L. Prophylactic inoculation against hay fever. The Lancet. 1911;**177**:1572-1573

[42] Freeman J, Noon L. Further observation on the treatment of hayfever by hypodermic inoculation of pollen vaccine. Lancet. 1911;**2**:814-817

[43] Black JH. The oral administration of pollen: Clinical report. The Journal of Laboratory and Clinical Medicine. 1928;**13**:709-713

[44] Rebien W, Wahn U, Puttonen E, Maasch HG. Comparative study of immunological and clinical efficacy of oral and subcutaneous hyposensitization. Allergologie. 1980;**3**:101-109

[45] Scadding GK, Brostoff J. Low dose sublingual therapy in patients with allergic rhinitis due to house dust mite. Clinical Allergy. 1986;**16**(5):483-491

[46] Tari MG, Mancino M, Monti G. Efficacy of sublingual immunotherapy in patients with rhinitis and asthma due to house dust mite. A double blind study. Allergologia et Immunopathologia. 1990;**18**:277-284. [PMID: 2097894]

[47] Bagnasco M, Mariani G, Passalacqua G, Motta C, Bartolomei M, Falagiani P, Mistrello G, Canonica GW. Absorption and distribution kinetics of the major Parietaria judaica allergen (Par j 1) administered by noninjectable routes in healthy human beings. The Journal of Allergy and Clinical Immunology. 1997;**100**(1):122-129

[48] Malling H, Weeke B. Immunotherapy. Position paper of the European Academy of Allergy and Clinical Immunology. Allergy. 1993;**48**(Suppl 14):9-35

[49] Malling HJ, Abreu-Nogueira J, Alvarez-Cuesta E, Bjorksten B, Bousquet J, Caillotet D, et al. Position paper of the European Academy of Allergy and Clinical Immunology on local immunotherapy. Allergy. 1998;**53**:933-944. [PMID: 9821472]

[50] Di Rienzo V, Pagani A, Parmiani S, Passalacqua G, Canonica GW. Post-marketing surveillance study on the safety of sublingual immunotherapy in children. Allergy. 1999;**54**:1110-1113. [PMID: 10536891]

[51] Lombardi C, Gargioni S, Melchiorre A, Passalacqua G. Safety of sublingual immunotherapy in adults: A post marketing surveillance study. Allergy. 2001;**56**:889-892. [PMID: 11576079]

[52] Bousquet J, Lockey R, Malling HJ, World Health Organization. Position paper. Allergen immunotherapy: Therapeutical vaccines for allergic diseases. Allergy. 1998;**53**:41-42

[53] Wilson D, Torres-Lima M, Durham S. Sublingual immunotherapy for allergic rhinitis. Cochrane Database of Systematic Reviews 2003, Issue 2. Art. No.: CD002893. DOI: 10.1002/14651858.CD002893

[54] Živković Z, Djurić-Filipović I, Živanović S. Current issues on sublingual allergen-specific immunotherapy in children with asthma and allergic rhinitis. Srpski Arhiv Za Celokupno Lekarstvo. 2016;**144**(5-6):345-350

[55] Penagos M, Passalacqua G, Compalati E, Baena-Cagnani CE, Orozco S, Pedroza A, et al. Metaanalysis of the efficacy of sublingual immunotherapy in the treatment of allergic asthma in pediatric patients, 3 to 18 years of age. Chest. 2008;**133**:599-609. [PMID: 17951626]

[56] Calderón M, Brandt T. Treatment of grass pollen allergy: Focus on a standardized grass allergen extract—Grazax®. Therapeutics and Clinical Risk Management. 2008;**4**(6): 1255-1260

[57] Dahl R, Kapp A, Colombo G, de Monchy JG, Rak S, Emminger W, Rivas MF, Ribel M, Durham SR. Efficacy and safety of sublingual immunotherapy with grass allergen tablets for seasonal allergic rhinoconjunctivitis. The Journal of Allergy and Clinical Immunology. 2006;**118**(2):434-440

[58] Dahl R, Kapp A, Colombo G, de Monchy JG, Rak S, Emminger W, Riis B, Grønager PM, Durham SR. Sublingual grass allergen tablet immunotherapy provides sustained clinical benefit with progressive immunologic changes over 2 years. The Journal of Allergy and Clinical Immunology. 2008;**121**(2):512-518.e2. Epub 2007 Dec 26

[59] Dahl R, Stender A, Rak S. Specific immunotherapy with SQ standardized grass allergen tablets in asthmatics with rhinoconjunctivitis. Allergy. 2006;**61**(2):185-190

[60] Durham SR, Riis B. Grass allergen tablet immunotherapy relieves individual seasonal eye and nasal symptoms, including nasal blockage. Allergy. 2007;**62**(8):954-957

[61] Nelson H, Blaiss M, Nolte H, Würtz SØ, Andersen JS, Durham SR. Efficacy and safety of the SQ-standardized grass allergy immunotherapy tablet in mono- and polysensitized subjects. Allergy. 2013;**68**:252-255. DOI: 10.1111/all.12074. [PMID: 23205670]

[62] Marogna M, Spadolini I, Massolo A, Zanon P, Berra D, Chiodini E, Canonica WG, Passalacqua G. Effects of sublingual immunotherapy for multiple or single allergens in polysensitized patients. Annals of Allergy, Asthma & Immunology. 2007;**98**(3):274-280

[63] Marogna M, Spadolini I, Massolo A, Canonica GW, Passalacqua G. Long-lasting effects of sublingual immunotherapy according to its duration: A 15-year prospective study. The Journal of Allergy and Clinical Immunology. 2010;**126**(5):969-975. DOI: 10.1016/j.jaci.2010.08.030. [PMID: 20934206]

[64] Marogna M, Bruno M, Massolo A, Falagiani P. Long-lasting effects of sublingual immunotherapy for house dust mites in allergic rhinitis with bronchial hyperreactivity A long-term (13-year) retrospective study in real life. International Archives of Allergy and Immunology. 2007; **42**(1):70-8.

[65] Holt PG, Sly PD, Sampson HA, Robinson P, Loh R, Lowenstein H, et al. Prophylactic use of sublingual allergen immunotherapy in high-risk children: A pilot study. The Journal of Allergy and Clinical Immunology. 2013;**132**(4):991-993.e1. DOI: 10.1016/j.jaci.2013.04.049. [PMID: 23768574]

[66] Shamji MH, Durham SR. Mechanisms of immunotherapy to aeroallergens. Clinical & Experimental Allergy. 2011;**41**:1235-1246. DOI: 10.1111/j.1365-2222.2011.0380. [PMID: 21762223]

[67] Szépfalusi Z, Bannert C, Ronceray L, Mayer E, Hassler M, Wissmann E, et al. Preventive sublingual immunotherapy in preschool children: First evidence for safety and pro-tolerogenic effects. Pediatric Allergy and Immunology. 2015;**25**:788-795. DOI: 10.1111/pai.12310. [PMID: 25406682]

[68] Eng PA, Borer-Reinhold M, Heijnen IAFM, Gnehm HPE. Twelve year follow-up after discontinuation of preseasonal grass pollen immunotherapy in childhood. Allergy. 2006;**61**:198-201. [PMID: 16409196]

[69] Malling HJ, Montagut A, Melac M, Patriarca G, Panzner P, Seberova E, et al. Efficacy and safety of 5-grass pollen sublingual immunotherapy tablets in patients with different clinical profiles of allergic rhinoconjunctivitis. Clinical & Experimental Allergy. 2009;**39**(3):387-393. DOI: 10.1111/j.1365-2222.2008.03152.x. [PMID: 19134019]

[70] Linneberg A. The allergic march in early childhood and beyond. Clinical & Experimental Allergy. 2008;**38**:1419-1421. DOI: 10.1111/j.1365-2222.2008.03063.x. [PMID: 18631352]

[71] Burgess JA, Lowe AJ, Matheson MC, Varigos G, Abramson MJ, Dharmage SC. Does eczema lead to asthma? Journal of Asthma. 2009;**46**:429-436. DOI: 10.1080/02770900902846356. [PMID: 19544160]

[72] Zivkovic Z, Cerovic S, Vukasinovic Z, Jocic-Stojanovic J. News in treatment of childhood asthma. Srpski Arhiv Za Celokupno Lekarstvo. 2009;**137**(9-10):558-561. DOI: 10.2298/SARH0910558Z. [PMID: 19950768]

[73] Bousquet J, Schünemann HJ, Zuberbier T, Bachert C, Baena-Cagnani CE, Bousquet PJ, et al. Development and implementation of guidelines in allergic rhinitis-an ARIA-GA2LEN paper. Allergy. 2010;**65**:1212-1221. DOI: 10.1111/j.1398-9995.2010.02480.x. [PMID: 20887423]

[74] Cerovic S, Zivkovic Z, Milenkovic B, Jocic-Stojanovic J, Opancina-Bajec A, Vukasinovic Z. The Serbian version of the pediatric asthma quality of life questionnaire in daily

practice. Journal of Asthma. 2009;**46**:936-939. DOI: 10.3109/02770900903265812. [PMID: 19905922]

[75] Živković Z, Radić S, Cerović S, Vukašinović Z. Asthma school program in children and their parents. World Journal of Pediatrics. 2008;**4**:267-273. DOI: 10.1007/s12519-008-0049-z. [PMID: 19104890]

[76] Calderon MA, Demoly P, Gerth van Wijk R, Bousquet J, Sheikh A, Frew A, et al. EAACI: A European Declaration on Immunotherapy. Designing the future of allergen specific immunotherapy. Clinical and Translational Allergy. 2012;**2**:20. Available from: http:// www. ctajournal.com/content/2/1/20

[77] Djuric-Filipovic I, Caminati M, Kostic G, Filipovic DJ, Zivkovic Z. An update of allergen specific sublingual immunotherapy in children with asthma and allergic rhinitis. World Journal of Pediatrics. 2016;**2**(3):283-290

[78] Caminati M, Rita Dama A, Djuric I, Montagni M, Schiappoli M, Ridolo E, Senna G, Canonica GW. Incidence and risk factors for subcutaneous immunotherapy anaphylaxis: The optimization of safety. Expert Review of Clinical Immunology. 2014;11:**1-1311**(2):233-45

[79] Lin SY, Erekosima N, Kim JM, Ramanathan M, Suarez-Cuervo C, Chelladurai Y, et al. Sublingual immunotherapy for the treatment of allergic rhinoconjuntivits and asthma. The Journal of the American Medical Association. 2013;**309**:1278-1288

[80] Bachert C, Canonica GW, Bufe A. SIT: Efficacy depends on product, not on route of application. Pediatric Allergy and Immunology. 2012;**23**:401

[81] Nichani JR, de Carpentier J. Safety of sublingual grass pollen immunotherapy after anaphylaxis. Journal of Laryngology & Otology. 2009;**123**(6):683-684

[82] Aydogan M, Eifan AO, Keles S, Akkoc T, Nursoy MA, Bahceciler NN, et al. Sublingual immunotherapy in children with allergic rhinoconjunctivitis mono-sensitized to house-dust-mites: A double-blind-placebo-controlled randomised trial. Respiratory Medicine. 2013;**107**:1322-1329

[83] Blaiss M, Maloney J, Nolte H, Gawchik S, Yao R, Skoner DP. Efficacy and safety of timothy grass allergy immunotherapy tablets in North American children and adolescents. The Journal of Allergy and Clinical Immunology. 2011;**127**:64-71, 71.e1-4

[84] Rodriguez-Perez N, Ambriz-Moreno AJ, Canonica GW, Penagos M. Frequency of acute systemic reactions in patients with allergic rhinitis and asthma treated with sublingual immunotherapy. Annals of Allergy, Asthma & Immunology. 2008;**101**:304-310

[85] Antico A, Pagani M, Crema A. Anaphylaxis by latex sublingual immunotherapy. Allergy. 2006;**61**:1236-1237

[86] Blazowski L. Anaphylactic shock because of sublingual immunotherapy overdose during third year of maintenance dose. Allergy. 2008;**63**:374

[87] de Groot H, Bijl A. Anaphylactic reaction after the first dose of sublingual immunotherapy with grass pollen tablet. Allergy. 2009;**64**:963-964

[88] Drachenberg KJ, Urban E, Proll S, Woroniecki SR. Sublingual specific immunotherapy for adults and children: A post marketing survey. Allergologia et Immunopathologia. 2004;**32**:76-81

[89] Agostinis F, Tellarini L, Canonica GW, Falagiani P, Passalacqua G. Safety of sublingual immunotherapy with a monomeric allergoid in very young children. Allergy. 2005;**60**:133

[90] Di Rienzo VD, Minelli M, Musarra A, Sambugaro R, Pecora S, Canonica WG, et al. Post marketing survey on the safety of sublingual immunotherapy in children below the age of 5 years. Clinical & Experimental Allergy. 2005;**35**:560-564

[91] Fiocchi A, Pajno G, La Grutta S, Pezzuto F, Incorvaia C, Sensi L, et al. Safety of SLIT in children aged 3 to 7 years. Annals of Allergy, Asthma & Immunology. 2005;**95**:254-258

[92] Mellerup MT, Han GW, Poulsen LK, Malling H. Safety of allergen-specific immunotherapy. Relation between dosage regimen, allergen extract, disease and systemic side-effects during induction treatment. Clinical & Experimental Allergy. 2000;**30**:1423-1429

[93] Agostinis F, Foglia C, Landi M, Cottini M, Lombardi C, Canonica GW, et al. The safety of sublingual immunotherapy with one or multiple pollen allergens in children. Allergy. 2008;**63**:1637-1639

[94] Pajno GB, Vita D, Parmiani S, Caminiti L, La Grutta S, Barberio G. Impact of sublingual immunotherapy on seasonal asthma and skin reactivity in children allergic to Parietaria pollen treated with inhaled fluticasone propionate. Clinical & Experimental Allergy. 2003;**33**:1641-1647

[95] De Castro G, Zicari AM, Indinnimeo L, Tancredi G, di Coste A, Occasi F, et al. Efficacy of sublilngual immunotherapy on allergic asthma in children's real life. European Review for Medical and Pharmacological Sciences. 2013;**17**:2225-2231

[96] Caminati M, Dama A, Schiappoli M, Senna G. Balancing efficacy against safety in sublingual immunotherapy with inhalant allergens: What is the best approach? Expert Review of Clinical Immunology. 2013;**9**:937-947

[97] Calderón MA, Simons FE, Malling HJ, Lockey RF, Moingeon P, Demoly P. Sublingual allergen immunotherapy: Mode of action and its relationship with the safety profile. Allergy 2012;**67**:302-311

[98] Senna G, Ridolo E, Calderon M, Lombardi C, Canonica GW, Passalacqua G. Evidence of adherence to immunotherapy. Current Opinion in Allergy and Clinical Immunology. 2009;**9**:544-548

[99] Pajno GB, Caminiti L, Crisafulli G, Barberi S, Landi M, Aversa T, et al. Adherence to sublingual immunotherapy in preschool children. Pediatric Allergy and Immunology. 2012;**23**:688-689

[100] Senna G, Caminati M, Canonica GW. Safety and tolerability of sublingual immunotherapy in clinical trials and real life. Current Opinion in Allergy and Clinical Immunology. 2013;**13**:656-662

[101] Juniper EF, Guyatt GH. Development and testing of a new measure of health status for clinical trias in rhinoconjunctivitis. Clinical & Experimental Allergy. 1991; **21**:77-83

[102] Ciprandi G, Cadario G, Valle C, Ridolo E, Verini M, Di Gioacchino M, et al. Sublingual immunotherapy in polysensitized patients: Effect on quality of life. The Journal of Investigational Allergology and Clinical Immunology. 2010;**20**:274-279

[103] Bousquet J, Scheinmann P, Guinnepain MT, Perrin-Fayolle M, Sauvaget J, Tonnel AB, et al. Sublingual swallow immunotherapy (SLIT) in patients with asthma due to house dust mites; a double blind placebo controlled study. Allergy. 1999;**54**:249-260

[104] Khinchi MS, Poulsen LK, Carat F, André C, Hansen AB, Malling HJ. Clinical efficacy of sublingual and subcutaneous birch pollen allergen-specific immunotherapy: A randomized, placebo-controlled, double-blind, double-dummy study. Allergy. 2004;**59**:45-53

[105] Frew AJ, Smith HE. Sublingual immunotherapy. The Journal of Allergy and Clinical Immunology. 2001;**107**:441-444

[106] Francis JN, James LK, Paraskevopoulos G, Wong C, Calderon MA, Durham SR, et al. Grass pollen immunotherapy: IL-10 induction and suppression of late responses precedes IgG4 inhibitory antibody activity. The Journal of Allergy and Clinical Immunology. 2008;**121**:1120-1125

[107] Aslam A, Chan H, Warrell DA, Misbah S, Ogg GS. Tracking antigenspecific T-cells during clinical tolerance induction in humans. PLoS One. 2010;**5**:e11028

[108] Suarez-Fueyo A, Ramos T, Galan A, Jimeno L, Wurtzen PA, Marin A. Grass tablet sublingual immunotherapy downregulates the TH2 cytokine response followed by regulatory T-cell generation. The Journal of Allergy and Clinical Immunology. 2014;**133**:130-138

[109] Akdis M, Burgler S, Crameri R, Eiwegger T, Fujita H, Gomez E, et al. Interleukins, from 1 to 37, and interferon-gamma: Receptors, functions, and roles in diseases. The Journal of Allergy and Clinical Immunology. 2011;**127**:701-721

[110] Josefowicz SZ, Lu LF, Rudensky AY. Regulatory T cells: Mechanisms of differentiation and function. Annual Review of Immunology. 2012;**30**:531-564

[111] Cavkaytar O, Akdis CA, Akdis M. Modulation of immune responses by immunotherapy in allergic diseases. Current Opinion in Pharmacology. 2014;**17C**:30-37

[112] van de Veen W, Stanic B, Yaman G, Wawrzyniak M, Söllner S Akdis DG, et al. IgG4 production is confined to human IL-10-producing regulatory B cells that suppress antigen-specific immune responses. The Journal of Allergy and Clinical Immunology. 2013;**131**:1204-1212

[113] Deniz G, van de Veen W, Akdis M. Natural killer cells in patients with allergic diseases. The Journal of Allergy and Clinical Immunology. 2013;**132**:527-535

[114] Jacobsen L, Wahn U, Bilo MB. Allergen-specific immunotherapy provides immediate, long-term and preventive clinical effects in children and adults: The effects of immunotherapy can be categorised by level of benefit—The centenary of allergen specific subcutaneous immunotherapy. Clinical and Translational Allergy. 2012;**2**:8

[115] Stylianou E, Ueland T, Borchsenius F, Michelsen AE, Øvstebø R, Eirik T, Mollnes T, Skjønsberg OH, Aukrust P. Specific allergen immunotherapy: Effect on IgE, IgG4 and chemokines in patients with allergic rhinitis. Scandinavian Journal of Clinical and Laboratory Investigation. 2016;**76**(2):118-127

[116] Shamji MH, James LK, Durham SR. Serum immunologic markers for monitoring allergen-specific immunotherapy. Immunology and Allergy Clinics of North America. 2011;**31**:311-323

[117] Niederberger V, Horak F, Vrtala S, Spitzauer S, Krauth MT, Valent P, et al. Vaccination with genetically engineered allergens prevents progression of allergic disease. Proceedings of the National Academy of Sciences of the United States of America. 2004;**101**:14677-14682

[118] Valenta R, Niespodziana K, Focke-Tejkl M, Marth K, Huber H, Neubauer A, et al. Recombinant allergens: What does the future hold? The Journal of Allergy and Clinical Immunology. 2011;**127**:860-864

[119] Lupinek C, Wollmann E, Baar A, Banerjee S, Breiteneder H, Broecker BM, et al. Advances in allergen-microarray technology for diagnosis and monitoring of allergy: The MeDALL allergen-chip. Methods. 2013;**66**:106-119

[120] Valenta R, Campana R, Marth K, van Hage M. Allergen-specific immunotherapy: From therapeutic vaccines to prophylactic approaches. Journal of Internal Medicine. 2012;**272**:144-157

[121] Hafner R, Salapatek A, Patel D, Larche M, Laidler P. Validation of peptide immunotherapy as a new approach in the treatment of allergic rhinoconjunctivitis: The clinical benefits of treatment with Amb a 1-derived T cell epitopes. The Journal of Allergy and Clinical Immunology. 2012;**129**:AB368

[122] Senti G, Crameri R, Kuster D, Johansen P, Martinez-Gomez JM, Graf N, et al. Intralymphatic immunotherapy for cat allergy induces tolerance after only 3 injections. The Journal of Allergy and Clinical Immunology. 2012;**129**:1290-1296

[123] Senti G, von Moos S, Tay F, Graf N, Sonderegger T, Johansen P, et al. Epicutaneous allergen-specific immunotherapy ameliorates grass pollen-induced rhinoconjunctivitis: A double-blind, placebo-controlled dose escalation study. The Journal of Allergy and Clinical Immunology. 2012;**129**:128-135

[124] Akdis CA. Therapies for allergic inflammation: Refining strategies to induce tolerance. Nature Medicine. 2012;**18**:736-749

[125] Wenzel SE. Asthma phenotypes: The evolution from clinical to molecular approaches. Nature Medicine. 2012;**18**:716-725

[126] Papadopoulos NG, Agache I,Bavbek S, Bilo BM, Braido F, Cardona V, et al. Research needs in allergy: An EAACI position paper, in collaboration with EFA. Clinical and Translational Allergy. 2012;**2**:21

[127] Ballow M, Akdis CA, Casale TB, Wardlaw AJ, Wenzel SE, Ballas Z, et al. Immune response modifiers in the treatment of asthma: A PRACTALL document of the American Academy of Allergy, Asthma & Immunology and the European Academy of Allergy and Clinical Immunology. The Journal of Allergy and Clinical Immunology. 2012;**130**:311-324

Chapter 7

Strategies to Study T Cells and T Cell Targets in Allergic Disease

Véronique Schulten

Additional information is available at the end of the chapter

http://dx.doi.org/10.5772/intechopen.68923

Abstract

Type I allergy is an immunoglobulin E (IgE)-mediated chronic disease. As such, disease diagnosis and identification of targeted allergens are primarily based on specific IgE reactivity. Over the past decades, the contribution of T cells in allergy pathogenesis has been extensively studied. T cells are not only significant for the onset and maintenance of allergic disease but likely also play a key role for the induction of tolerance by allergen-specific immunotherapy (AIT). Due to the complexity of allergic T cell responses, epitopes have only been thoroughly mapped for the most dominant and prevalent allergens. Recently developed laboratory approaches enable us to perform thorough peptide screens, identifying T cell epitopes in known and novel allergenic targets, irrespective of their IgE reactivity. Monitoring allergen-specific T cells and their phenotype will provide insights into disease manifestation and progression on a molecular level.

However, performing such experiments in the clinic is not feasible. The definition of dominant T cell epitopes will allow us to create a tool to assess allergen-specific T cells in the context of different disease severities, such as rhinitis, asthma, and/or immunotherapy which will likely hold the key for improved diagnostic, biomarkers, and even novel therapeutic approaches.

Keywords: allergy, T cells, Th2, IgE, epitope

1. Introduction

Type I allergy is an immunoglobulin E (IgE)-mediated chronic disease. As such, disease diagnosis and identification of targeted allergens are primarily based on specific IgE reactivity. Specifically, clinical practices for the diagnosis of allergic disease are most commonly based on skin prick testing [1], which typically involves pricking the skin with a needle or pin containing a small amount of allergen [2]. A second diagnostic test is commonly performed in vitro for allergen-specific immunoglobulin E (IgE), which can accurately evaluate and quantify the presence or absence of IgE specific for the whole allergen extract or single protein components [3].

The importance of IgE in mediating allergic disease, especially immediate-type reactions occurring within minutes of exposure to the allergen, is evident. However, the involvement of allergen-specific T cells and their pathological role in mediating late-phase reactions [4, 5] is often underappreciated. Allergenic proteins are defined based on their ability to bind IgE and the frequency of allergic patients harboring specific IgE antibodies to a given allergen [6, 7]. The potential of an allergenic protein to induce T cell reactivity is mostly not taken into account when classifying a protein as an allergen. Over the past decades, however, the contribution of T cells, specifically T helper 2 (Th2) cells, in mediating the pathogenesis of allergy has been extensively studied [8]. Immunological studies have shown that T cells play a key role early on, before allergic disease is even established. Susceptible individuals initially exposed to allergen mount a dominant Th2 response, resulting in the production of type 2 cytokines, such as IL-4 and IL-13. These cytokines along with a direct physical interaction of T and B cells occurring between CD40L expressed on the surface of the activated T cell and CD40 constitutively expressed by B cells provide the signal for B cells to undergo antibody class switching and produce allergen-specific IgE [9, 10], a process referred to as allergic sensitization. Subsequently, IgE molecules now present in high abundance bind with high affinity to Fcε receptors expressed on granulocytes, where they are cross-linked by allergen molecules upon reexposure, leading to mediator release and immediate-type symptoms, such as urticarial, allergic rhinitis, and conjunctivitis. Immediate-type reactivity is followed by late-phase reactions, which typically occur several hours/days after exposure to allergen. During the late-phase reaction, the affected tissue is infiltrated by Th2 cells and other inflammatory cells including eosinophils and neutrophils, which secrete high levels of cytokines, such as IL-4 and IL-5 to promote inflammation [8].

T cells are not only significant for the onset and maintenance of allergic disease but likely also play a key role for the induction of tolerance, which can be achieved by allergen-specific immunotherapy (AIT) and is the only curative treatment for allergic disease to date. Due to the complexity of human T cell responses against allergens, epitopes have only been thoroughly mapped for the most dominant and prevalent allergens. Recently developed laboratory approaches enable us to perform thorough peptide screens, which achieve the identification and immunological characterization of T cell epitopes in known and novel allergenic targets, irrespective of their IgE reactivity [11, 12]. Mapping of T cell epitopes is of high importance: it greatly facilitates the detection, immunological analysis, and phenotypic characterization of allergen-specific T cells in patients suffering from allergic or asthmatic disease as well as providing a tool to monitor the efficacy of allergen-specific immunotherapy (AIT) treatment. While allergen extracts can also be used to stimulate allergen-specific T cell responses, extracts are not standardized resulting in great variability of allergen content between extract batches [13–15], and endotoxin content is often not monitored [16]. Further, processing and presentation of a large number of peptides present in extract limit the abundance of peptides that represent dominant T cell epitopes. It has been reported that allergen-specific T cells in tissues and peripheral blood are of very low frequency [17, 18], ranging from approximately 10^{-5} to 10^{-3} CD4+ T cells, outside or within the pollen season, respectively. The rarity of these cells poses a great challenge for immune mechanistic studies designed to probe how allergic pathology or tolerance induction during AIT administration is orchestrated. The identification of dominant T cell epitopes can therefore be of great importance not only to understand the molecular entities targeted by allergen-specific T cells but also to use them as a tool to detect, isolate, and characterize allergen-specific T cells.

The frequency of patients harboring IgE responses against a specific allergen is most often known and used for classification of the allergen as a minor or major allergen in a respective population [19, 20]. In contrast, T cell epitope data is only available for a small subset of allergens listed by the International Union of Immunological Society (IUIS) database [12]. The relative lack of data on allergen T cell epitopes is likely due to the highly complex nature of T helper cell responses in allergic disease, which makes it a difficult system for immunological studies. Moreover, allergen-specific T cells occur at a very low frequency in the peripheral blood [18], making them hard to detect and isolate. Nevertheless, immunological studies on the allergic T cell response in humans have become of growing importance over the last years. Accordingly, new technologies and concepts have been developed to overcome the challenges of studying allergen-specific T cell responses, map single epitopes, and phenotypically characterize peptide-specific T cells to gain more insights into how T cells contribute to the pathology of allergy and asthma.

2. Challenges of T cell epitope mapping

The identification of T cell epitopes from major allergens is an important goal in allergy research. A critical step for inducing a T cell response against an allergen is the recognition of allergen-derived peptides. These peptides are presented to the T cell by antigen-presenting cells (APCs), such as dendritic cells or monocytes, in the context of major histocompatibility complex (MHC) class II molecules, which are constitutively expressed by APCs. MHC class II molecules are encoded by three different loci, designated HLA DR, DQ, and DP. Each of these three loci is extremely polymorphic adding a high degree of complexity, which has to be accounted for in the design of T cell epitope mapping strategies [21].

2.1. Overlapping versus predicted peptide

To identify T cell epitopes in allergy, the most diligent approach involves testing overlapping peptides that span the entire sequence of the allergen of interest. For this setup, the entire allergen sequence is broken down into short peptides, typically 12–20 amino acids in length, overlapping by 9–12 residues. These peptides are then tested for their ability to induce T cell reactivity, using peripheral blood mononuclear cells (PBMCs) from allergic patients, often after in vitro expansion with allergen or allergen extract [22, 23]. Peptides that elicit T cell reactivity, as measured by cytokine production, proliferation, or upregulation of T cell activation markers, are reported as T cell epitopes. T cell epitope mapping using overlapping peptides is a very thorough approach, designed to identify any possible T cell-activating region within the allergen. However, mapping peptides for bigger allergens or even multiple allergens can add up to a very high number of peptides to test, also increasing the amount of blood needed for screening and the cost and effort associated. To make large-scale epitope identification more feasible, an approach was developed that involves preselection of peptides based on their ability to bind human MHC class II molecules. MHC molecules have a relatively broad specificity for peptide binding. The three-dimensional structure forms a binding cleft that can bind peptides of varying length, typically ranging from 15 to 25 amino acids [24, 25]. The capacity of a peptide ligand to bind MHC class II molecules can be quantitatively measured directly by assessing its ability to inhibit the binding of a radiolabeled probe peptide to purified MHC molecules [26]. However, such experiments are labor intensive and expensive; therefore, computational tools are continuously being developed to model and predict peptide-MHC binding [27, 28]. Using predicted peptide binding as a preselection criterion to decrease the number of peptides to screen for T cell epitope identification is less thorough than using overlapping peptides and may therefore increase the risk of missing T cell-reactive peptides. However, it has been reported that it is a reliable approach to identify the vast majority of T cell epitopes [28, 29], and it has been successfully used in several allergen systems, including Timothy grass [11], German cockroach [30], house dust mite [31], and others [32], to perform large-scale epitope identification studies. Therefore, the decision between using overlapping and predicted peptides is likely dictated by the size and number of allergens studied as well as the amount of cells available from the clinical cohort.

2.2. Allergen-specific T cell frequencies

Another challenging aspect of T cell epitope identification in allergy is the low frequency of allergen-specific T cells. A study that evaluated the ex vivo frequency of T cells specific for Fel d 1, the major cat allergen, reported that the percentage of CD4+ T cells specific for a single Fel d 1 epitope ranged from 0.014 to 0.0003% in allergic individuals [33]. Another study, focused on Mugwort allergy, reported an ex vivo frequency of peptide-specific T cells of 0–0.029% in allergic cohort [34]. In a third study, performed with cells from patients allergic to Timothy grass, the authors reported epitope-specific T cell frequencies of 0.6–0.75% of the total CD4+ T cell subset [35], with a modest increase in frequencies detected during grass pollen season. The rarity of allergen-specific T cells poses a great challenge for epitope identification, as it will require the T cell reactivity assay to reliably detect a few single cells that respond to the peptide among several thousands of CD4+ T cells. In addition, a large amount of blood volume would be required to screen a given number of peptides. To bypass this problem, in vitro expansion cultures are performed, in which lymphocytes from allergic individuals are cultured over a few days or weeks with allergen extract or recombinant allergen protein to which the donor is allergic. The allergen in the culture will activate and stimulate the few antigen-specific T cells present in the culture, causing them to proliferate. Typically, recombinant human IL-2 is added in limiting dilution in regular intervals after the first few days of culture to increase proliferation of allergen-specific cells, which have upregulated their IL-2 receptor during cell activation. Over time, allergen-specific cells, which were rare in the starting culture, become highly enriched due to antigen-specific stimulation and proliferation. After several days, the cells can be harvested in screened for T cell reactivity in response to restimulation with single peptides. In the presence of allergen or whole allergen extract, allergen peptide-specific T cells will have expanded and are now present in high abundance, making them easily detectable after restimulation with single peptides. T cell reactivity I response to a peptide can be measured by a variety of assays, most commonly using proliferation, cytokine production, or upregulation of activation marker as a readout [22, 36, 37]. This method is extremely useful to expand very rare antigen-specific CD4+ populations. However, one major limitation associated with in vitro expansion culture is that it changes the original phenotype of the cells. Therefore, it cannot be performed if an immunological characterization of the phenotype of the antigen-specific cells is desired. Analyses designed to investigate the genetic expression profile have to be performed on cells isolated directly ex vivo, which is difficult due to their aforementioned rarity in the peripheral blood.

3. Immunological characterization of allergen-specific T cells

There are several approaches to isolate allergen-specific cells ex vivo for subsequent downstream immunological profiling using technologies, such as RNA or TCR sequencing. These technologies have become of increasing importance in areas, such as biomarker discovery or developing tools to monitor the efficacy of allergen-specific immunotherapy.

3.1. MHC tetramer assay

The use of MHC tetramer reagents to detect antigen-specific T cells is a well-established technique that allows detection and further downstream analysis of allergen-specific cells on a single cell level. The tetramer molecule is made up of a fluorescently labeled, centric streptavidin molecule bound to biotin-labeled MHC molecules, which are loaded with a peptide known to be a T cell epitope to form the peptide-MHC complex (**Figure 1A**) [38]. The resulting tetramer can then be used as a reagent to bind T cells that are specific for both, the MHC type and peptide used in the tetramer (**Figure 1B**). Cells that are specific and bind the tetramer are now fluorescently labeled and can be detected and isolated using a flow cytometer. There are several applications for tetramer staining all based on the premise that it allows the detection of single antigen-specific cells, even if they occur at low frequency. In vaccinology, tetramers are often used to track frequencies of peptide-specific T cells in the blood before and after vaccination or boost. Similarly, in allergy, tetramers have been used to quantify numbers of specific T cells as a variable of allergen season [35], allergen-specific immunotherapy [39], and disease status [34, 40]. In addition, tetramer staining can be combined with other methodologies to perform more detailed immunological characterization of allergen-specific T cells. Simultaneous assessment of cell proliferation, cytokine production, or activation can provide

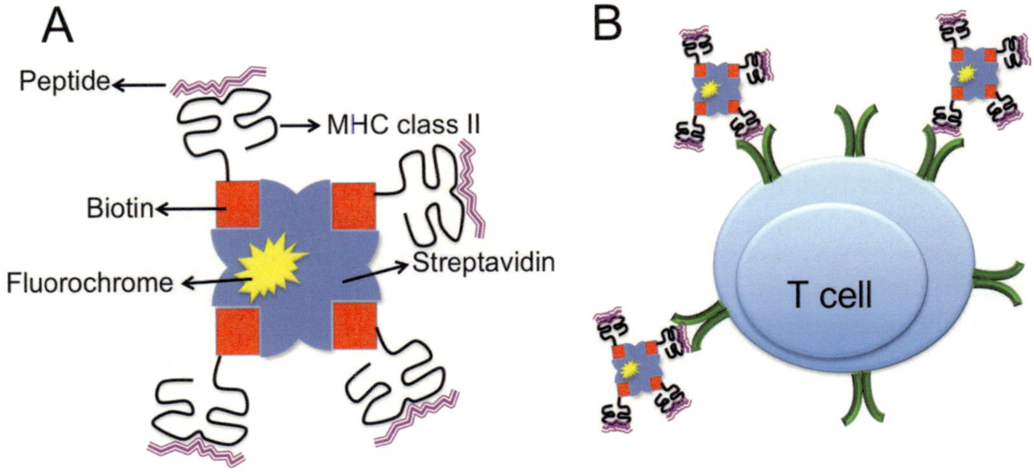

Figure 1. (A) Schematic representation of the structural complex of a MHC class II tetramer and (B) binding of tetramer molecules to the peptide-specific T cell via the T cell receptor (TCR).

functional information in addition to knowing the peptide specificity and MHC restriction of the cell. Tetramer reagents can even be used for T cell epitope mapping. This approach involves loading empty MHC molecules with pools of mixtures of overlapping peptides from the allergen of interest, each pool typically containing 5–10 peptides. These tetramers are then screened with PBMC that have been cultured with the allergen of interest. Pools that positively detect T cell populations are deconvoluted into single peptides, which are loaded onto MHC molecules individually and then analyzed to identify single epitopes. Tetramers that return positive stainings automatically provide a population of T cells with a known MHC restriction and antigen specificity, which can be sorted by fluorescence-activated cell sorting (FACS) allowing downstream analysis of phenotype and genotype. This approach has successfully been used in allergy to identify T cell epitopes [41].

MHC tetramer assays represent a revolution for the study of antigen-specific T cells, providing an efficient way to directly visualize, quantify, phenotype, and isolate T cells of interest. Yet, this technology is also associated with disadvantages and limitations. The construction of tetramer reagents is not trivial and requires an advanced level of expertise. Production and purification of high-quality MHC molecules are labor intensive, and only a subset of MHC alleles expressed by humans is available as tetramer. Further, the use of tetramers requires existing knowledge about the HLA restriction of the peptide of interest. In allergy, many dominant T cell epitopes are highly promiscuous, meaning they are restricted by multiple alleles, which makes finding their restriction more difficult. Determining the HLA restriction of given peptides can be done experimentally, for example, by inhibition with locus-specific antibodies [32]. This method, however, only identifies the restricting locus. Data from HLA-binding assays can also be a useful tool to narrow down the possible restriction [42]. Another approach designed to determine HLA restriction at the allele level involved the use of single HLA class II-transfected cell lines [43]; however, a large panel of cell lines is required to determine restrictions in multiple donors due to the heterogeneity of HLA types in a given population. As an alternative to the experimental approaches, which are labor intensive and technically challenging, a bioinformatical prediction tool was developed. This tool uses T cell response data in an HLA-typed population to infer HLA restriction by genetic association [44]. Although this tool streamlines the prediction of HLA restriction, it still requires experimental T cell response data and an HLA-typed population large enough to make significant predictions possible.

The use of tetramer reagents requires preexisting knowledge about the HLA restrictions for a given peptide as well as the HLA type of the donor sample. Acquiring this information can be costly and labor intensive, making this approach less feasible for certain studies.

3.2. Cytokine capture assay

The isolation of antigen-specific cells based on cytokine production used to be complicated by the fact that T cells positive for cytokine production were detected by intracellular cytokine staining, which involved fixation and permeabilization of the cell. Fixed cells are no longer alive and can therefore not be used for downstream applications that require live cells, and even isolation of DNA or RNA from fixed cells is somewhat more complex than from live cells. A new approach that captures cytokines on the cell surface immediately after secretion was developed to allow detection and isolation of viable cells that secrete cytokines in response to antigen stimulation. In this protocol, cells are pre-labeled with a "catch reagent," a divalent complex consisting of a CD45-specific monoclonal antibody conjugated to monoclonal antibody directed against the cytokine of interest. The anti-CD45 antibody will bind to CD45 molecules expressed on the T cell surface and effectively coat the cell (**Figure 2**). Subsequently, cells are stimulated with antigen, and any cytokine produced will be bound to the cytokine-specific antibody conjugated to anti-CD45 immediately after secretion. Detection of cytokine-positive cells is achieved by using a fluorescent-labeled detection antibody with the same cytokine specificity but recognizing a different epitope from the catch reagent antibody (**Figure 2**). If the antigen-specific T cell population is extremely rare, which is often the case in allergy and asthma, an enrichment step can be performed. To further enrich antigen-specific cells before flow cytometric analysis or isolation, microbeads conjugated to monoclonal antibodies specific for the respective fluorophore used in the experiment can be used to label cells, followed by magnetic column enrichment [35]. After cells are labeled and the enrichment step has been performed if desired, viable cells can be analyzed and isolated by flow cytometry, facilitating downstream applications, such as further culture assays or DNA/RNA extraction for sequencing analysis. A potential limitation of this assay is the bias introduced by isolating cells based on production of a single cytokine. Often, cytokine production in response to allergens is heterogeneous, and cells produce different levels of different cytokines, such as IL-4, IL-5, IL-13, and sometimes IFNg. Detection of allergen-specific cells based on production of a single cytokine will likely lead to an underrepresentation of allergen-specific cells, since cells producing a different cytokine will not be detected.

3.3. Cell activation assays

Another hallmark of antigen-specific T cells is the upregulation of activation markers in response to antigen stimulation. Therefore, these activation markers can be targeted with

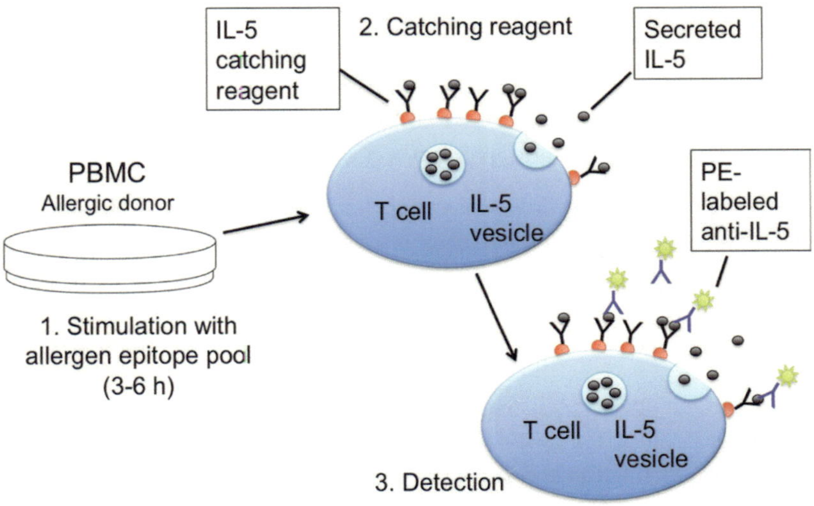

Figure 2. A schematic representation of the methodology involved for a cytokine capture assay, using IL-5 as representative cytokine.

fluorescent antibodies to detect antigen or allergen-specific cells. The challenge of this approach is to identify activation markers that are specific and highly expressed to allow reliable detection of allergen-specific T cells even at low frequency. One molecule that has become very popular for such an application is CD154, also known as CD40 ligand (CD40L). CD154 is a member of the tumor necrosis factor (TNF) superfamily and found to be primarily expressed on activated T cells, making it very specific. It acts as a co-stimulatory molecule, binding to CD40 on antigen-presenting cells, which can lead to several downstream events depending on the target cell type. Several studies designed to study allergen-specific effector cells in cohorts suffering from allergy, asthma, or who have been treated with AIT have successfully applied this methodology to immunologically characterize and isolate allergen-specific T cells ex vivo [37, 45]. The caveat of using CD154 as a selection marker for activated, allergen-specific T cells is that it is also typically stained intracellularly. In humans, CD154 molecules expressed on the cell surface quickly become unstable, making a large number of CD154 expressing cells undetectable. Therefore, this assay typically involves fixation and permeabilization to allow intracellular staining of CD154, making downstream applications less feasible.

As an alternative to CD154, other activation markers, such as Ox40 and CD25 have also been used to detect and isolate antigen-specific cells after short-term antigen stimulation [46]. The main advantage of this approach is that both Ox40 and CD25 are stably expressed on the cell surface and therefore cells can be detected and isolated in viable form without the need of fixation or permeabilization. However, CD25 is also strongly expressed by regulatory T cells, irrespective of activation; therefore, gating of Ox40 and CD25 double-positive cells has to be performed with great accuracy, and the inclusion of a third marker, such as PDL-1 may be considered to avoid contamination of nonspecific T cells.

3.4. Proliferation assays

The identification of antigen-specific cells based on the proliferative response to antigenic stimulation is perhaps the most classical approach and has been widely used for several applications including T cell epitope mapping, phenotypic characterization, T cell response kinetics, and others. In the past, the classic method to detect cell proliferation in response to allergen stimulation involved the addition of radioactive nucleoside, 3H-thymidine, to the culture, which would be automatically incorporated into new strands of chromosomal DNA during mitotic cell division. Subsequently, proliferation was assessed by measuring the radioactivity in DNA recovered from the cell sample using a scintillation beta-counter. Though this technology is still used in some laboratories, proliferation is now more commonly detected by flow cytometry. One common approach is the staining of cells with a special fluorescent dye, which is then diluted through each cell division. This decrease in the concentration of the dye can be visualized by flow cytometry. Another approach is to stain stimulated cells with antibodies targeting markers associated with proliferation, such as Ki67. The measure of proliferation in response to antigen stimulation is straightforward and inexpensive. The greatest caveat associated with using proliferation as a readout for antigen-specific reactivity is the relatively high rate of false positivity due to bystander activation. A study designed to directly compare the use of tetramer staining reagents versus allergen-induced proliferation for the detection of allergen-specific T cells found that while tetramers had a relatively low rate of sensitivity, cells identified based on proliferation contained extremely high fractions of bystander cells [34], making this approach more suitable if an enriched population is sufficient for the study rather than a desire for a pure antigen-specific population.

4. Targeting T cells in allergen-specific immunotherapy

Allergy and asthma are debilitating diseases that are most commonly treated using pharmacotherapy which are designed to improve the symptoms but not the cause of disease. To date, the only disease-modifying therapy available is allergen-specific immunotherapy (AIT). First administered over a century ago [47], AIT has been widely demonstrated to be a clinically effective treatment, inducing immunological tolerance and improvement of clinical symptoms beyond the time of treatment [48]. Despite its favorable duration of efficacy, a considerable effort is invested to improve current AIT protocols. Allergen-specific immunotherapy with whole extract can be associated with IgE-mediated adverse reactions that result from the patient's allergen-specific IgE molecules being cross-linked by the allergen present in the extract used for treatment, triggering degranulation and immediate-type reactions. The occurrence of such adverse events and the need for extended treatment periods that last several years can have a negative impact on treatment compliance. For this reason, researchers have strived to find a treatment that targets T cells and circumvents potential IgE reactivity. Removal of IgE epitopes, thereby eliminating the risk of IgE cross-linking, is one obvious approach. There are a variety of methods to achieve this goal, some of which have been evaluated in clinical trials.

4.1. Peptide immunotherapy

One extensively pursued approach for AIT focused on T cells while omitting IgE epitopes is called peptide immunotherapy, where instead of using whole allergen extract, allergic patients are treated with a mixture of short, synthetic peptides that constitute the major T cell epitopes of the allergen the patient is allergic to. The clinical efficacy of peptide immunotherapy has been demonstrated in several Phase IIb double-blind, placebo-controlled trials [49, 50]. A significant reduction in symptoms, measured as the total rhinoconjunctivitis symptom score (TRSS), was observed following the administration of only eight intradermal injections of the peptide formulation. In this study, TRSS levels remained suppressed both at the 1- and 2-year follow-up time point [51]. The immunological mechanisms by which peptide immunotherapy induces tolerance are not yet fully understood. However, studies have reported a downregulation of pathological type 2 cell responses and a concomitant increase in regulatory signals, such as the production of IL-10 in the periphery. Further, significant increases in IFNg-producing Th1 cells and CD25+ cells have been reported. The induction of IgG4-blocking antibodies, which are believed to contribute to clinical efficacy by occupying the allergen-binding sites, thereby preventing IgE-allergen binding, is a hallmark event during conventional AIT with allergen extract. Interestingly, increased levels of IgG4 are rarely observed, probably due to the lack of conformational B cell epitopes decreasing the likelihood of B cell stimulation and resulting IgG production. Therefore, though modulatory events on the cellular level appear to be broadly similar to those believed to occur during extract-based AIT, humoral responses may be more distinct. Although peptide immunotherapy has been shown to be clinically effective, it is also associated with challenges that need to be addressed. The route of administration has been debated, and the clinical effects seem to be very sensitive to dosing. Lower doses may not induce tolerance due to lack of potency for induction of regulatory T cells, while too high dose may stimulate and expand pathogenic Th2 cells. The selection of peptides is also a factor of consideration. Typically, mixtures used for peptide immunotherapy include between 5 and 10 peptides. However, epitope specificities can be very heterologous in a given population, and therefore the selection may not be straightforward. The consideration of these factors and others make the development of peptide immunotherapy challenging at times.

4.2. Fragmented allergens

Another approach of AIT that was designed to target T cells while bypassing IgE binding to avoid IgE-mediated side effects is the generation of fragmented allergens. This approach was tested using the major birch pollen allergen, Bet v 1, as a model. The fragmentation of the allergen involved its division into non-IgE-binding fragments, which retain their T cell reactivity. Birch pollen allergic patients were then vaccinated with these hypoallergenic derivatives in a double-blind, placebo-controlled study. This vaccination was found to reduce cutaneous sensitivity, improve symptoms, and significantly reduce rises in birch-specific IgE levels during season in the active group compared to placebo [52]. However, immunological mechanisms and long-term efficacy were not evaluated.

5. Concluding remarks

Allergic disease severity is very poorly understood. The degree of symptom manifestation, such as asthma versus rhinitis can often not be explained by allergen-specific IgE titers. There is a dire need for better diagnostics and biomarkers that will help us evaluate treatment options and disease prognosis. Gaining a better understanding of the immunological events on a cellular level may have a tremendous impact on how we treat patients in the clinic. Monitoring allergen-specific T cells and their phenotype will provide insights into disease manifestation and progression on a molecular level. However, performing such experiments in the clinic is not feasible. The definition of dominant T cell epitopes will allow us to create a tool to assess allergen-specific T cells in the context of different disease severities, such as rhinitis, asthma, and/or immunotherapy which will likely hold the key for improved diagnostic, biomarkers, and even novel therapeutic approaches.

Acknowledgements

This work has been funded with federal funds from the National Institute of Allergy and Infectious Diseases, National Institutes of Health, Department of Health and Human Services, under the grant number U19AI100275.

Author details

Véronique Schulten

Address all correspondence to: veronique@lji.org

La Jolla Institute for Allergy and Immunology, La Jolla, CA, USA

References

[1] Ryan MW, Marple BF, Leatherman B, Mims JW, Fornadley J, Veling M, Lin SY. Current practice trends in allergy: Results of a united states survey of otolaryngologists, allergist-immunologists, and primary care physicians. International Forum of Allergy & Rhinology. 2014;**4**:789-795

[2] Bernstein IL, Li JT, Bernstein DI, Hamilton R, Spector SL, Tan R, Sicherer S, Golden DB, Khan DA, Nicklas RA, Portnoy JM, Blessing-Moore J, Cox L, Lang DM, Oppenheimer J, Randolph CC, Schuller DE, Tilles SA, Wallace DV, Levetin E, Weber R, American Academy of Allergy A, Immunology, American College of Allergy A, Immunology. Allergy diagnostic testing: An updated practice parameter. Annals of allergy, Asthma

& Immunology: Official Publication of the American College of Allergy, Asthma, & Immunology. 2008;**100**:S1-S148

[3] Szeinbach SL, Barnes JH, Sullivan TJ, Williams PB. Precision and accuracy of commercial laboratories' ability to classify positive and/or negative allergen-specific IgE results. Annals of Allergy, Asthma & Immunology: Official Publication of the American College of Allergy, Asthma, & Immunology. 2001;**86**:373-381

[4] Barata LT, Ying S, Meng Q, Barkans J, Rajakulasingam K, Durham SR, Kay AB, IL-4- and IL-5-positive T lymphocytes, eosinophils, and mast cells in allergen-induced late-phase cutaneous reactions in atopic subjects. The Journal of Allergy and Clinical Immunology. 1998;**101**:222-230

[5] Huh JC, Strickland DH, Jahnsen FL, Turner DJ, Thomas JA, Napoli S, Tobagus I, Stumbles PA, Sly PD, Holt PG. Bidirectional interactions between antigen-bearing respiratory tract dendritic cells (DCs) and T cells precede the late phase reaction in experimental asthma: DC activation occurs in the airway mucosa but not in the lung parenchyma. The Journal of Experimental Medicine. 2003;**198**:19-30

[6] Andersson K, Lidholm J. Characteristics and immunobiology of grass pollen allergens. International Archives of Allergy and Immunology. 2003;**130**:87-107

[7] Basketter DA, Kimber I. Assessing the potency of respiratory allergens: Uncertainties and challenges. Regulatory Toxicology and Pharmacology: RTP. 2011;**61**:365-372

[8] Romagnani S. Regulation of the development of type 2 T-helper cells in allergy. Current Opinion in Immunology. 1994;**6**:838-846

[9] Spriggs MK, Armitage RJ, Strockbine L, Clifford KN, Macduff BM, Sato TA, Maliszewski CR, Fanslow WC. Recombinant human CD40 ligand stimulates B cell proliferation and immunoglobulin E secretion. The Journal of Experimental Medicine. 1992;**176**:1543-1550

[10] Gauchat JF, Gascan H, de Waal Malefyt R, de Vries JE. Regulation of germ-line epsilon transcription and induction of epsilon switching in cloned EBV-transformed and malignant human B cell lines by cytokines and CD4+ T cells. Journal of Immunology. 1992;**148**:2291-2299

[11] Schulten V, Greenbaum JA, Hauser M, McKinney DM, Sidney J, Kolla R, Lindestam Arlehamn CS, Oseroff C, Alam R, Broide DH, Ferreira F, Grey HM, Sette A, Peters B. Previously undescribed grass pollen antigens are the major inducers of T helper 2 cytokine-producing T cells in allergic individuals. Proceedings of the National Academy of Sciences of the United States of America. 2013;**110**:3459-3464

[12] Schulten V, Oseroff C, Alam R, Broide D, Vijayanand P, Peters B, Sette A. The identification of potentially pathogenic and therapeutic epitopes from common human allergens. Annals of Allergy, Asthma & Immunology: Official Publication of the American College of Allergy, Asthma, & Immunology. 2013;**110**:7-10

[13] Duffort O, Palomares O, Lombardero M, Villalba M, Barber D, Rodriguez R, Polo F. Variability of Ole e 9 allergen in olive pollen extracts: Relevance of minor allergens in immunotherapy treatments. International Archives of Allergy and Immunology. 2006; **140**:131-138

[14] Meyer CH, Bond JF, Chen MS, Kasaian MT. Comparison of the levels of the major allergens Der p I and Der p II in standardized extracts of the house dust mite, Dermatophagoides pteronyssinus. Clinical and Experimental Allergy: Journal of the British Society for Allergy and Clinical Immunology. 1994;**24**:1041-1048

[15] Vailes L, Sridhara S, Cromwell O, Weber B, Breitenbach M, Chapman M. Quantitation of the major fungal allergens, Alt a 1 and Asp f 1, in commercial allergenic products. The Journal of Allergy and Clinical Immunology. 2001;**107**:641-646

[16] Trivedi B, Valerio C, Slater JE. Endotoxin content of standardized allergen vaccines. The Journal of Allergy and Clinical Immunology. 2003;**111**:777-783

[17] Sager N, Feldmann A, Schilling G, Kreitsch P, Neumann C. House dust mite-specific T cells in the skin of subjects with atopic dermatitis: Frequency and lymphokine profile in the allergen patch test. The Journal of Allergy and Clinical Immunology. 1992;**89**:801-810

[18] Wambre E, Van Overtvelt L, Maillere B, Humphreys R, von Hofe E, Ferhat L, Ebo D, Moingeon P, Single cell assessment of allergen-specific T cell responses with MHC class II peptide tetramers: Methodological aspects. International Archives of Allergy and Immunology. 2008;**146**:99-112

[19] Rossi RE, Monasterolo G, Monasterolo S. Measurement of IgE antibodies against purified grass-pollen allergens (Phl p 1, 2, 3, 4, 5, 6, 7, 11, and 12) in sera of patients allergic to grass pollen. Allergy. 2001;**56**:1180-1185

[20] Tovey ER, Baldo BA. Detection of house dust mite allergens and frequency of IgE binding following electroblotting and enzyme immunoassay. International Archives of Allergy and Applied Immunology. 1985;**76**:82-85

[21] Schulten V, Peters B, Sette A. New strategies for allergen T cell epitope identification: Going beyond IgE. International Archives of Allergy and Immunology. 2014;**165**:75-82

[22] Oseroff C, Sidney J, Kotturi MF, Kolla R, Alam R, Broide DH, Wasserman SI, Weiskopf D, McKinney DM, Chung JL, Petersen A, Grey H, Peters B, Sette A. Molecular determinants of T cell epitope recognition to the common Timothy grass allergen. Journal of Immunology. 2010;**185**:943-955

[23] Zulehner N, Nagl B, Briza P, Roulias A, Ballmer-Weber B, Zlabinger GJ, Ferreira F, Bohle B, Characterization of the T-cell response to Dau c 1, the Bet v 1-homolog in carrot. Allergy. 2017;**72**:244-251

[24] Sette A, Ceman S, Kubo RT, Sakaguchi K, Appella E, Hunt DF, Davis TA, Michel H, Shabanowitz J, Rudersdorf R, et al. Invariant chain peptides in most HLA-DR molecules of an antigen-processing mutant. Science. 1992;**258**:1801-1804

[25] O'Brien C, Flower DR, Feighery C. Peptide length significantly influences in vitro affinity for MHC class II molecules. Immunome Research. 2008;**4**:6

[26] Sidney J, Southwood S, Moore C, Oseroff C, Pinilla C, Grey HM, Sette A. Measurement of MHC/peptide interactions by gel filtration or monoclonal antibody capture. Current Protocols in Immunology. 2013; Chapter 18: Unit 18.3.1-18.3.26.

[27] Wang P, Sidney J, Kim Y, Sette A, Lund O, Nielsen M, Peters B. Peptide binding predictions for HLA DR, DP and DQ molecules. BMC Bioinformatics. 2010;**11**:568

[28] Wang P, Sidney J, Dow C, Mothe B, Sette A, Peters B. A systematic assessment of MHC class II peptide binding predictions and evaluation of a consensus approach. PLoS Computational Biology. 2008;**4**:e1000048

[29] Moutaftsi M, Peters B, Pasquetto V, Tscharke DC, Sidney J, Bui HH, Grey H, Sette A. A consensus epitope prediction approach identifies the breadth of murine T(CD8+)-cell responses to vaccinia virus. Nature Biotechnology. 2006;**24**:817-819

[30] Dillon MB, Schulten V, Oseroff C, Paul S, Dullanty LM, Frazier A, Belles X, Piulachs MD, Visness C, Bacharier L, Bloomberg GR, Busse P, Sidney J, Peters B, Sette A. Different Bla-g T cell antigens dominate responses in asthma versus rhinitis subjects. Clinical and Experimental Allergy: Journal of the British Society for Allergy and Clinical Immunology. 2015;**45**:1856-1867

[31] Oseroff C, Christensen LH, Westernberg L, Pham J, Lane J, Paul S, Greenbaum J, Stranzl T, Lund G, Hoof I, Holm J, Wurtzen PA, Meno KH, Frazier A, Schulten V, Andersen PS, Peters B, Sette A. Immunoproteomic analysis of house dust mite antigens reveals distinct classes of dominant T cell antigens according to function and serological reactivity. Clinical and Experimental Allergy: Journal of the British Society for Allergy and Clinical Immunology. 2016;**47**(4): 577-592.

[32] Oseroff C, Sidney J, Vita R, Tripple V, McKinney DM, Southwood S, Brodie TM, Sallusto F, Grey H, Alam R, Broide D, Greenbaum JA, Kolla R, Peters B, Sette A. T cell responses to known allergen proteins are differently polarized and account for a variable fraction of total response to allergen extracts. Journal of Immunology. 2012;**189**:1800-1811

[33] Kwok WW, Roti M, Delong JH, Tan V, Wambre E, James EA, Robinson D. Direct ex vivo analysis of allergen-specific CD4+ T cells. The Journal of Allergy and Clinical Immunology. 2010;**125**:1407-1409 e1

[34] Van Hemelen D, Mahler V, Fischer G, Fae I, Reichl-Leb V, Pickl W, Jutel M, Smolinska S, Ebner C, Bohle B, Jahn-Schmid B. HLA class II peptide tetramers vs allergen-induced proliferation for identification of allergen-specific CD4 T cells. Allergy. 2015;**70**:49-58

[35] Hinz D, Seumois G, Gholami AM, Greenbaum JA, Lane J, White B, Broide DH, Schulten V, Sidney J, Bakhru P, Oseroff C, Wambre E, James EA, Kwok WW, Peters B, Vijayanand P, Sette A. Lack of allergy to timothy grass pollen is not a passive phenomenon but associated with the allergen-specific modulation of immune reactivity. Clinical and Experimental Allergy: Journal of the British Society for Allergy and Clinical Immunology. 2016;**46**:705-719

[36] Schulten V, Nagl B, Scala E, Bernardi ML, Mari A, Ciardiello MA, Lauer I, Scheurer S, Briza P, Jurets A, Ferreira F, Jahn-Schmid B, Fischer GF, Bohle B. Pru p 3, the nonspecific lipid transfer protein from peach, dominates the immune response to its homolog in hazelnut. Allergy. 2011;**66**:1005-1013

[37] Bacher P, Heinrich F, Stervbo U, Nienen M, Vahldieck M, Iwert C, Vogt K, Kollet J, Babel N, Sawitzki B, Schwarz C, Bereswill S, Heimesaat MM, Heine G, Gadermaier G, Asam C, Assenmacher M, Kniemeyer O, Brakhage AA, Ferreira F, Wallner M, Worm M, Scheffold A. Regulatory T cell specificity directs tolerance versus allergy against aeroantigens in humans. Cell. 2016;**167**:1067-1078 e16

[38] Sims S, Willberg C, Klenerman P, MHC-peptide tetramers for the analysis of antigen-specific T cells. Expert Review of Vaccines. 2010;**9**:765-774

[39] Wambre E, DeLong JH, James EA, Torres-Chinn N, Pfutzner W, Mobs C, Durham SR, Till SJ, Robinson D, Kwok WW. Specific immunotherapy modifies allergen-specific CD4(+) T-cell responses in an epitope-dependent manner. The Journal of Allergy and Clinical Immunology. 2014;**133**:872-879, e7

[40] Wambre E, Bonvalet M, Bodo VB, Maillere B, Leclert G, Moussu H, Von Hofe E, Louise A, Balazuc AM, Ebo D, Hoarau C, Garcia G, Van Overtvelt L, Moingeon P. Distinct characteristics of seasonal (Bet v 1) vs. perennial (Der p 1/Der p 2) allergen-specific CD4(+) T cell responses. Clinical and Experimental Allergy: Journal of the British Society for Allergy and Clinical Immunology. 2011;**41**:192-203

[41] DeLong JH, Simpson KH, Wambre E, James EA, Robinson D, Kwok WW. Ara h 1-reactive T cells in individuals with peanut allergy. The Journal of Allergy and Clinical Immunology. 2011;**127**:1211-1218, e3

[42] Arlehamn CS, Sidney J, Henderson R, Greenbaum JA, James EA, Moutaftsi M, Coler R, McKinney DM, Park D, Taplitz R, Kwok WW, Grey H, Peters B, Sette A. Dissecting mechanisms of immunodominance to the common tuberculosis antigens ESAT-6, CFP10, Rv2031c (hspX), Rv2654c (TB7.7), and Rv1038c (EsxJ). Journal of Immunology. 2012;**188**:5020-5031

[43] McKinney DM, Southwood S, Hinz D, Oseroff C, Arlehamn CS, Schulten V, Taplitz R, Broide D, Hanekom WA, Scriba TJ, Wood R, Alam R, Peters B, Sidney J, Sette A. A strategy to determine HLA class II restriction broadly covering the DR, DP, and DQ allelic variants most commonly expressed in the general population. Immunogenetics. 2013;**65**:357-370

[44] Paul S, Dillon MB, Lindestam Arlehamn CS, Huang H, Davis MM, McKinney DM, Scriba TJ, Sidney J, Peters B, Sette A. A population response analysis approach to assign class II HLA-epitope restrictions. Journal of Immunology. 2015;**194**:6164-6176

[45] Campbell JD, Buchmann P, Kesting S, Cunningham CR, Coffman RL, Hessel EM. Allergen-specific T cell responses to immunotherapy monitored by CD154 and intracellular cytokine

expression. Clinical and Experimental Allergy: Journal of the British Society for Allergy and Clinical Immunology. 2010;**40**:1025-1035

[46] Dan JM, Lindestam Arlehamn CS, Weiskopf D, da Silva Antunes R, Havenar-Daughton C, Reiss SM, Brigger M, Bothwell M, Sette A, Crotty S. A cytokine-independent approach to identify antigen-specific human germinal center T follicular helper cells and rare antigen-specific CD4+ T cells in blood. Journal of Immunology. 2016;**197**:983-993

[47] Noon L. Prophylactic inoculation against hay fever. Lancet. 1911;**1**:1572-1573

[48] Durham SR, Walker SM, Varga EM, Jacobson MR, O'Brien F, Noble W, Till SJ, Hamid QA, Nouri-Aria KT. Long-term clinical efficacy of grass-pollen immunotherapy. The New England Journal of Medicine. 1999;**341**:468-475

[49] Oldfield WL, Larche M, Kay AB. Effect of T-cell peptides derived from Fel d 1 on allergic reactions and cytokine production in patients sensitive to cats: A randomised controlled trial. Lancet. 2002;**360**:47-53

[50] Worm M, Lee HH, Kleine-Tebbe J, Hafner RP, Laidler P, Healey D, Buhot C, Verhoef A, Maillere B, Kay AB, Larche M. Development and preliminary clinical evaluation of a peptide immunotherapy vaccine for cat allergy. The Journal of Allergy and Clinical Immunology. 2011;**127**:89-97, e1-14 e7

[51] Patel D, Couroux P, Hickey P, Salapatek AM, Laidler P, Larche M, Hafner RP. Fel d 1-derived peptide antigen desensitization shows a persistent treatment effect 1 year after the start of dosing: A randomized, placebo-controlled study. The Journal of Allergy and Clinical Immunology. 2013;**131**:103-109, e1-7

[52] Niederberger V, Horak F, Vrtala S, Spitzauer S, Krauth MT, Valent P, Reisinger J, Pelzmann M, Hayek B, Kronqvist M, Gafvelin G, Gronlund H, Purohit A, Suck R, Fiebig H, Cromwell O, Pauli G, van Hage-Hamsten M, Valenta R. Vaccination with genetically engineered allergens prevents progression of allergic disease. Proceedings of the National Academy of Sciences of the United States of America. 2004;**101**(Suppl 2):14677-14682

Chapter 8

Gamma Radiation Effect on Allergenic Food

Marcia Nalesso Costa Harder, Valter Arthur and
Larissa Nalesso Costa Harder

Additional information is available at the end of the chapter

http://dx.doi.org/10.5772/intechopen.69581

Abstract

Food allergens are substances that cause an overreaction of the individual immune system of who consumes it. The importance of food allergy in the nutritional present context is increasing, and dietary habits and nutrient availability have rapidly transformed in function of access to consumers. There is no specific treatment for food allergies. It is necessary to stop eating the food. Studies with the use of nuclear radiation to minimize these effects have been performed. The absorption of electromagnetic radiation by the biological tissues that constitute the food produces a function of electronic excitability of the constituent molecules. An example of this reaction is with proteins leading to deamination, breaking peptides, aromatic residues formation, and so on. The extent of these reactions depends on the food conditions and substances that are contained in.

Keywords: ionizing radiation, food irradiation, food allergy

1. Introduction

The use of ionizing radiation was applied in foods given the discovery of radiation at the end of the nineteenth century, since several researches have been carried out in several follow-ups from this unique event for humanity.

Most of the studies on food irradiation describe about the use of technology in microbial control, including the effective and efficient mode of pathogen control, as well as the use to improved post-harvest products.

Mastro [1] explains that the food irradiation reduces the risk of foodborne diseases as has already been established by many studies, and the food thus treated maintains the nutritional value of macrocomponents and suffers loss of microcomponents as is the case with vitamins. The World Health Organization (WHO) has expressed its views on this, as well as jointly WHO, Food and Agriculture Organization (FAO) and the International Atomic Energy Agency (IAEA). For these international institutions, foods irradiated according to good manufacturing practices (GMP) are safe for consumption and suitable from the nutritional point of view. Irradiated foods are provided for astronauts for years and are the best option for immunosuppressed patients, as well as to meet the emergency food supply during natural disasters.

According to Prejean [2], food security is widely recognized as an increasingly significant public health problem worldwide. For him, regardless of its admitted effectiveness against foodborne pathogens, the employment of irradiation is still rare in the food industry, and the inquiry is as to why a technology that is extremely effective and safe by any scientific test would be greeted with such uncertainty by the food industry.

After exhaustive studies on this topic, recent research has found an alternative use for inosinate radiation using this technology to minimize the allergenic effects of food.

The EACCI [3] defines the allergy as a hypersensitivity reaction begun by immunological mechanisms. The sensitivity can be mediated by antibodies or by cells. In a large number of events, the antibody worthy of the symptoms belongs to the IgE isotype, and the organisms may be mentioned as suffering from an IgE-mediated allergy. Not every allergic response connected with IgE occurs in atopic individuals. In non-IgE-intervened allergy, the antibody may fit into the IgG isotype, for example, anaphylaxis caused by immune complexes holding dextran, as well as in the classical serum disease, previously referred to as type III reaction. Both immunoglobulin E (IgE) and immunoglobln G (IgG) can be found in allergic bronchopulmonary aspergillosis (ABPA). Allergic contact dermatitis is representative of allergic diseases mediated by lymphocytes.

As advocated by Taylor in the early 1980s, food allergy prevention can be achieved by altering dietary factors responsible for the sensitization and phenotypic expression of the disease. Since then, proteolytic enzyme hydrolysis of allergens and the development of recombinant food with modified DNA have been the hope in the elimination of protein allergens when compared to traditional processing methods [4]. However, these affirmations can be utilized only in limited foods [5].

For now, the structural change of food proteins by radiation was studied by Kume et al. [6], and this result revealed that ionizing radiation could modify antigenicity by the undoing or alteration of conformational and linear epitopes in food allergens [7, 8]. Recently, the complete abolition of intrinsic activity and loss of structural integrity with fragmentation and aggregation following wide-dose irradiation have been observed in several studies [5].

Because of these questions related before, the aim of this paper is to provide some insight into how the peaceful use of ionizing energy can contribute to improve the quality of life of people with some type of food allergy.

2. Ionizing radiation

Harder and Arthur [9] defined radiation as either the transmission or the emission of energy through a material medium or space in the form of particles or waves. Radiation is categorized as

http://dx.doi.org/10.5772/intechopen.69581

either nonionizing or ionizing. Nonionizing radiation does not have enough energy to completely remove an electron from a molecule or an atom and is ordinarily not harmful to living organisms. It consists of lower ultraviolet, visible light, infrared, microwaves, radio waves, or lower energy electromagnetic waves emitted by power suppliers or receivers for television or radio. By contrast, ionizing radiation does have the energy to liberate electrons from molecules and atoms transforming them into ions. Therefore, ionizing radiation consists of not only ions and atoms but also subatomic particles as well as electromagnetic waves on the high-energy end of the electromagnetic spectrum.

2.1. Gamma ray irradiation

The simplest form of irradiation is gamma ray irradiation. The origin of radiation is a radioactive element that sends protons in the gamma ray reach of the electromagnetic spectrum. Gamma ray photons have a higher recurrence (and hence, energy) than either ultraviolet or X-ray photons. It can permeate a target food to a depth of diverse feet and range of microbial contaminants anywhere within that reach. But it is simple on concept, because in addition to radiating gamma rays, many radioactive elements also produce alpha rays (helium nuclei), beta rays (high-energy electrons or positrons), and/or high-energy neutrons, so it is important to choose well the source of the radiation. Alternatively, they might decay into another radioactive substance that generates these other forms of radiation, but they are undesirable because they have the potential to make the target food radioactive. Gamma rays can be contained by immersion of the source in a sufficient quantity of water, and to prevent inadvertent gamma ray exposure, the source must be insulated from the outside world by several feet of concrete [2, 10].

2.2. E-beam irradiation

For the same authors, E-beam irradiation, even if it uses that identical term as gamma ray irradiation, is a fully different type of treatment. High-energy electron beams are made in an electron gun, a larger version of the cathode ray gun discovered in devices such as televisions and monitors. The electrons can be headed by a magnetic area to aim food. The term "irradiation" is indeed a misnomer, since the food is not stated to electromagnetic radiation or beta rays (electrons made by a radioactive source). Notwithstanding, the development has a resembling effect to that of gamma ray irradiation. E-beam irradiation demands protection as well, but nothing as the concrete box used in gamma ray irradiation. The drawback of the E-beam is its small penetration depth (about an inch), avoiding its use to many foods and restricting the amount of food that can be processed in volume.

2.3. X-ray irradiation

X-ray irradiation is a fairly new technique that matches many of the benefits of the other two processes. As gamma ray irradiation, X-ray irradiation consists of exhibiting food to high-energy photons with a long permeation depth. In this situation, nevertheless, bombarding a metal film with a high-energy electron beam yields the photons, permitting the radiation to be turned on and off. The apparatus is a more powerful version of the X-ray machines used in medical cabinets. The device still demands heavy safeguard, though the amount of protection required is less than that for gamma ray irradiation. No radioactive material or byproducts are used in, or outcome from, the process [2, 10].

3. Food radiation

The term "food irradiation" refers to any process that exposes food either to electromagnetic radiation or to high-energy particles [2].

Briefly, food radiation is the processing of foods by expounding them to a controlled quantity of ionizing energy for a particular number of times to attain determined technical objectives. Food is irradiated in a particular method facility where it is subject to gamma rays, electron beams, or X-rays. The food is strictly monitored to ensure that the precise dose or treatment levels are performed. When used in this way, irradiation is similar to pasteurization of milk, in that the good is left fresh but much more out of danger.

For Harder and Arthur [11], the principal lead of radiation use in food is a completely default of direct use of chemical elements that may leave residuum in treated food, making it unassured for consumption. Thus, ionizing radiation used in food attracted interest around the world from many organizations such as the IAEA, FAO, OECD (Organization for Economic Cooperation and Development), and WHO along with the participation of 24 countries in studies to untangle the modifications that are consequences of the use of radiation in the food.

Food radiation is ultimately about how much energy is adsorbed by the mark food. It is important to have a metering for what shot of radiation will be necessary independent of the quantity of food to be irradiated. Radiation doses are calculated in kiloGray (kGy). A portion of 1 kGy shows that the goal specimen receives 1000 J (metric units of energy, for short J) per kilogram of sample bulk. The result of radiation on microbes is measured by a dosage called the *D*-value [12].

The effectiveness of the treatment varies based on the type of radiation used (gamma ray, X-ray, or E-beam), the intensity of the radiation, and the purpose of the use in question.

Irradiation destroys injurious bacteria and other organisms, meat, poultry, and seafood, disinfests spices, spreads shelf-life of fresh fruits and vegetables, and also controls budding in tubers (e.g., potatoes) and bulbs (e.g., onions). As in illustration, a very short number of ionizing energy are worn to expunge insect pests from fruit; a little greater number is used on meat or poultry to destroy noxious bacteria, and notably higher number is used to fully sterilize food. Irradiation complements good manufacturing practices without compromising on food quality or nutrition [13].

For Harder and Arthur [9], there are three different irradiation methods (radappertization, radicidation, or radurization) used to inactivate microorganisms based on the severity of the process:

- Radappertization is the most severe of the three irradiation methods. With radappertization or sterilization of food, a dose of irradiation is applied that decreases the activity and number of living microbes (excludes viruses) to such a low level that there is no recognized method for detection. Doses required for radappertization are generally between 25 and 45 kGy [14, 15]. All foods—including eggs without shells in the form of egg white, yolk, or whole egg—subjected to radappertization must be parceled in hermetically sealed packets so that there is no recontamination of the product to the environment. Radappertization is popular for use in meat products such as chicken fillets and turkey breast. The National Aeronautics and Space Administration, the space agency of the United States, uses radappertization to prepare irradiated food for consumption of astronauts during space flights. The irradiated food products have no microbial viability, even at room temperature, provided the package is kept intact. All irradiated foods must have expiration dates regardless of whether the package is kept intact or not because prolonged storage causes chemical and physical changes in these products.

- Radicidation, similar to pasteurization, is the treatment of food with a sufficient dose of ionizing radiation to inactivate nonspore-forming bacteria in a way that the microorganisms are not detected by bacteriological methods normally used on processed foods. Doses required for radicidation are generally between 2 and 8 kGy [14, 15]. Examples of foods where radicidation is applied include juices, fresh meats, fresh pasta, and eggs.
- Radurization is the least severe of the three processes of irradiation with dosages in the range of 0.4–2.5 kGy. Radurization disinfects or sanitizes food and extends shelf-life by causing a reduction in the count of viable spoilage microorganisms. Examples of where radurization is used in foods include the following: (1) preventing the sprouting of bulbs and tubers, (2) preventing the deterioration of fruits and vegetables by fungi, (3) killing parasites, insects, and mites that infest food, and (4) slowing down the ripening of fruits. The delay in ripening and the shelf-life extension in fruits like bananas are great advantages as this fruit can ripen quickly without treatment. The use of radurization to delay the fruit-ripening process provides time for food distribution and exportation.

Other uses with ionizing radiation are the structural alteration of proteins, and it is being investigated as a means of reducing food allergies. Common food allergies in humans include milk β-lactoglobulin, shrimp tropomyosin, and egg albumin. Subjecting food to ionizing radiation changes the antigenicity of food by altering the physical and chemical structure of proteins leading to distortion of the protein's secondary and tertiary structures. Specifically, the epitope area of the food allergen can be modified or destroyed by gamma irradiation so that antibodies to the allergen should never be produced by the individual consuming the irradiated food [9, 16, 17].

The Food and Drug Administration (FDA) [18] treated that for all food submitted to food irradiation, the Radura symbol can be used to identify the process (**Figure 1**), which should be placed on irradiated food packages in many countries of the world. The Radura symbol originated from and was copyrighted by an irradiation food-processing facility located in Wageningen, Netherlands, in the 1960s. The then president Jan Leemhorst of the company called Gammaster recommended its use as an international label to be placed on irradiated food as long as manufacturers implemented appropriate quality parameters. The Radura symbol is listed in the Codex Alimentarius Standard on Labeling of Prepackaged Food. The FDA requires that foods that have been irradiated bear the "Radura" logo along with the statement "Treated with radiation" or "Treated by irradiation".

Figure 1. The Radura symbol.

3.1. Effects of food radiation

For food irradiation to be safe, radiolytic products (radiolytic products are chemicals created by the interaction of radiation with a substance such as food) must pose no danger for human consumers. Most of radiolytic goods are created by the radiation-rupturing molecular links in water, leaving spare radicals that in turn either recombine into water or interact with other chemicals. Other radiolytic products are created when complex protein molecules are broken into smaller ones. From the standpoint of radiation chemistry, then, irradiation is no more dangerous than cooking food, because radiolytic products formed by food irradiation are all found naturally in non-irradiated food, and the types of compounds formed by irradiation are identical to those formed during the cooking process [19].

Some vitamins, particularly thiamine, undergo an appreciable reduction when exposed to radiation. But in the totality of the diet, however, FDA determined that the average person's intake of these vitamins would be well above the recommended dietary allowance (RDA) [19].

Another situation from the food radiation is water radiolysis, or water broken by the ionizing radiation that forms analytes as H^+ and OH^-. From the water radiolysis, the formation of hydrogen peroxide has great significance in irradiated foods. Like all foods containing substances that can oxidize or reduce, many reactions can occur when foods containing water are irradiated [11].

3.2. Consumer acceptance and marketing of irradiated foods

Although irradiation cannot prevent primary contamination, it is the most effective tool available to significantly reduce or eliminate harmful bacteria in raw product. Food irradiation has the virtual to dramatically reduce the incidence of foodborne illness and has gained practically consentaneous aid or approbation from international and national medical, scientific, and public welfare organizations, also from food processors and associated industry groups. Numerous consumer studies clearly show that when given a choice and even a small amount

http://dx.doi.org/10.5772/intechopen.69581

of accurate information, consumers are not only willing to buy irradiated foods but also often prefer them over food treated by conventional means [13].

4. Food intolerance and allergies

Primary food sensitivities can be cloven into immunological and nonimmunological responses. The base of an unnatural immunological reaction after expenditure is a real food allergy or hypersensitivity. Primary sensitivities involving immunological retroactions are more piecemeal into IgE-mediated and non-IgE-mediated food allergies. The reactions are often noted as immediate hypersensitivity reactions, because the symptoms occur soon after ingesting the offending foods. Food allergens are defined as common food proteins (foods contain many proteins, but only a few of them are allergens). As in all people, the allergens are ingested, pass through the gut epithelium, and circulate in the blood; however, the immune system of some individuals reacts to these food allergens by manufacturing immunoglobulin E (IgE) [20].

5. Chemical and biological properties of food allergens

For Jedrychowski and Wichers [21], most of the allergens have a protein; they are usually glycoproteins dissolved in water and resistant to digestion. The immune system recognizes them, and as a result, specific IgEs are produced (type I allergy) or specific T-cell antigen receptors (TCRs) are produced (type IV allergy).

Harder et al. [11] treated the debate on the effect of radiation in proteins formed on the study of the radiation chemistry of amino acids. Started responses with hydrated electrons are the main route in the radiolysis of amino acids and proteins. When proteins are irradiated in the attendance of water, all of the retroactions that are possible with amino acids are also practicable with proteins holding these amino acids. With 20 component amino acids and proteins with three reactive kinds of water radiolysis, many complicated interactions are practical. Further, the effects are exercised by the spatial shape of the protein current, determined by hydrogen links, disulfide links, hydrophobic links, and ionic links. Lonely, amino acids, which are likely to attack by radicals when irradiated, are less susceptible when they are part of the protein structure and they are more or less inaccessible to responses with radicals. Another factor that probably contributes to the increased force compared with the protein-isolated amino acid sequence is owing to a greater or lesser hardness of the spatial structure of the protein; radicals created as a result of irradiation molecule are safe in the stance and have a high chance of recombination.

The authors also said that a great proportion of radiant energy laid up in irradiated proteins seemingly promotes denaturation, and modifies in secondary and tertiary current, before the destruction of the amino acid components. This denaturation is much less longer than that caused by warmth. This is because sterilizing radiation in food for much time housing combines with warm treatment. Enzymes are more sensible to warmth.

6. Application of gamma irradiation for inhibition of food allergy

According to Byun et al. [16], the amount of intact allergens in an irradiated solution can be reduced by gamma irradiation depending upon the dose. This situation occurs because that in the epitopes on the allergens can be structurally altered by radiation treatment and that the irradiation technology can be applied to reduce allergenicity of allergic foods.

Kume et al. [6] observed the structural modification of food proteins by radiation, and these results have indicated that ionizing radiation could change antigenicity by the destruction or modification of antibody-binding epitopes in food antigens/allergens.

7. Effect of irradiation on allergenicity of different food products

Food irradiation objective is the inactivation of microorganisms and through this to prolong the shelf-life. As side effect, this technology influences the food allergenicity.

The process of irradiating proteins with high dose besides inactivation of microorganisms induced the production of protein aggregates and degraded fragments with reactivity to the specific antibodies.

One example is the research that Vaz et al. [22] conducted. Studies on *Sebastiania jacobinensis* bark lectin found that high doses of gamma irradiation (above 1 kGy) induced a significant loss of activity of this protein. There were apparent changes in the hydrophobic surface. Gamma irradiation caused protein misfolding and aggregation.

After these reports, other research developed within the effect of irradiation on allergenicity of different food products thematic has been subsequently listed.

8. Eggs

For egg proteins, Lee et al. (2005) produced cakes containing layer of egg white that were gamma-irradiated with 10 or 20kGy in study promoted by them. The ovalbumin present decreased its allergenicity by irradiation and processing. Egg white irradiated for reducing the egg allergy could be used for producing a safer cake [23]. And then, Lee et al. [24] treated hen egg ovomucoid at basic pH irradiated at 10 kGy, heated at 100°C for 15 min, or both treatments were applied. The combination of irradiation and heating was very effective in reducing the amount of intact ovomucoid regardless of the pH condition. For Kume and Matsuda [7], the principle of the effect can be demonstrated in case of ovalbumin and bovine serum albumin in solution (0.2% in 0.01 M phosphate buffer, pH 7.4). These proteins were irradiated with a high dose of the order of 8 kGy (units for intensity characterization of ionization by gamma irradiation). This process besides inactivation of microorganisms induced the production of protein aggregates and degraded fragments with reactivity to the specific antibodies. The main part of conformation-dependent reactivity, spatial antigenic structure (conformational epitope), was lost, but some antigenicity persisted.

In their study, Kim et al. [25] was carried out to evaluate the changes in the allergenic and antigenic properties of hen's egg albumin (ovalbumin) with the combination of heat and gamma irradiation treatment. They found that the ovalbumin's capacity to connect to mouse lgG modified upon heating at 167°F and its capacity to connect to egg-allergic IgE modified upon heating at 176°F. The ELISAs introduced that egg-allergic IgE did not identify ovalbumin very well when warmish at ≥176°F, while mouse lgG maintained better activity under these requirements specimen treated by irradiation followed by warming. For that, these consequences demonstrate that allergies induced by ovalbumin could be effectively decreased by the blend of warm and gamma irradiation treatment.

Lee et al. [24] in their study evaluated the effect of a treatment combining gamma radiation and heating on the allergenic properties of hen's egg ovomucoid under basic pH conditions. They observed that the concentration of unimpaired ovomucoid reduced with irradiation or warming, and the fee of the reduction was larger for a basic pH requirement than for the physiological requirement. Ultimately, they concluded that the blend of irradiation and heating was very effective in reducing the amount of intact ovomucoid regardless of the pH condition. After treatment, the renovation of the pH to 7.4 did not affect the concentration of ovomucoid. The results of this study indicate that a combination of irradiation and warming might be an effective way for decreasing egg hypersensitivity resulting from ovomucoid.

9. Milk

Milk proteins allergen was studied by Lee et al. [26] who found that bovine alpha-casein and beta-lactoglobulin when irradiated changed their allergenicity and antigenicity. Probably, agglomeration of proteins was caused by the treatment.

In their study, Lee et al. [26] executed to assess the application of food irradiation technology as a way for decreasing milk allergies. In this scientific study, bovine alpha-casein and beta-lactoglobulin were used as milk proteins. The application of milk-hypersensitive patients' immunoglobulin E and rabbit IgGs individually made to bovine alpha-casein and beta-lactoglobulin, the shift of allergenicity and antigenicity of irradiated proteins was noted by competitive oblique enzyme-linked immunosorbent test.

For the authors, allergenicity and antigenicity of the irradiated proteins were modified unlike sides of the inhibition curves. The vanishing of the band on sodium dodecyl sulfate-polyacrylamide gel electrophoresis and the rise of the turbidity demonstrated that solubility of the proteins decreased by radiation, and it might be caused by agglomeration of the proteins. These results showed that epitopes on milk allergens were structurally changed by gamma irradiation.

10. Fish and seafood

Our research evaluated heat-stable protein that was secluded and processed with gamma radiation at 0, 1, 3, 5, 7, and 10 kGy in a requirement of solution (1 mg/ml) and fresh shrimp was irradiated too. The IgE-linking fee was decreased with an increasing dose. The principal allergenic protein was gone and the vestiges induced from coagulation showed up at a higher molecular weight zone as evidenced by a special test. The same results were received on proteins extracted from irradiated shrimp studied by Byun et al. [27].

Investigations on glutamic oxaloacetic transaminase, glutamic pyruvate transaminase, and rhodanese of both unirradiated and irradiated chub mackerel (*Rastrelliger neglectus*) have been carried out by Sofyan and Soedigdo [28]. They can be proved that glutamic oxaloacetic transaminase and glutamic pyruvate transaminase were more susceptible toward irradiation as compared to rhodanese. An irradiation dose of 4 kGy was able to inactivate glutamic oxaloacetic transaminase, glutamic pyruvate transaminase, and rhodanese for ca 50, 44, and 36%, respectively. Evidently, transaminase- as well as rhodanese-specific activities to spoiled fish were significantly lower ($P \leq 0.01$) than those of fresh fish. The residual glutamic oxaloacetic transaminase-, glutamic pyruvate transaminase-, and rhodanese-specific activities in spoiled fish were found to be about 35, 41, and 22%, respectively.

11. Wheat

Commercial gliadin powder and wheat flour were irradiated with doses between 2.2 and 12.8 kGy. Surprisingly, irradiated gliadin increased its allergenicity. Gliadin extracted from irradiated wheat flour exhibited higher immunoreactivity than pure gliadin irradiated with the same dose [29].

12. Conclusion

Regarding earlier explanation, we can conclude that the ionizing radiation is effective to control the allergenicity in food. But more studies are necessary to determine the chronic and acute doses, as well as the dose rate, pH, temperature, humidity, and other parameters that can influence the food characteristics.

Author details

Marcia Nalesso Costa Harder[1]*, Valter Arthur[2] and Larissa Nalesso Costa Harder[3]

*Address all correspondence to: marcia.harder@fatec.sp.gov.br

1 Technology College of Piracicaba "Dep. Roque Trevisan," Piracicaba, São Paulo, Brazil

2 Nuclear Energy Center in Agriculture—CENA/USP, Piracicaba, São Paulo, Brazil

3 State University Northern of Parana, Jacarezinho, Paraná, Brazil

References

[1] Mastro NL. Ionizing radiation for the promotion of adequate and healthy food. Vigilância Sanitária em Debate. 2015;**3**(2):114-121

[2] Prejean JE. Food Irradiation [Internet]. 2001. Available from: https://dash.harvard.edu/bitstream/handle/1/8846796/Prejeanpap.html?sequence=3 [Accessed: February 2017]

[3] EAACI. Definições em alergia [Internet]. 2017 [Updated: 2017]. Available from: http://www.eaaci.org/attachments/977_portuguese.htm [Accessed: February 2017]

[4] Nilsson C, Oman H, Harfast B. A case of allergy to cow's milk hydrolysate. Allergy. 1999; **54**:1322-1325

[5] Melo Vaz AF. Estabilidade estrutural e funcional de lectinas submetidas à irradiação gama: Potencial em alergia alimentar [thesis]. UFPE: UFPE; 2011. p. 141

[6] Kume T, Ishii T, Matsuda T. Immunochemical identification of irradiated chicken eggs. Journal of Science and Food Agriculture. 1994;**65**:1-4

[7] Kume T, Matsuda T. Changes in structural and antigenic properties of proteins by radiation. Radiation Physics and Chemistry. 1995;**46**:225-231

[8] Lee JW, Yook HS, Lee KH, Kim JH, Byun MW. Conformational changes of myosin by gamma irradiation. Radiation Physics and Chemistry. 2000;**58**:271-277

[9] Harder MNC, Arthur V. Effects of gamma radiation for microbiological control in eggs. In: Hester P, editor. Egg Innovation and Strategies for Improvement. 1st ed. Oxford: Elsevier Inc.; 2017. pp. 177-186

[10] Center for Disease Control (CDC). Frequently Asked Questions about Food Irradiation [Internet]. 1999 [Updated: 1999]. Available from: http://www.cdc.gov/ncidod/dbmd/diseaseinfo/foorirradiation.htm [Accessed: February 2017]

[11] Harder MNC, Arthur V, Arthur PB. Effect of ionizing radiation on food components. In: Caballero B, Finglas P, Toldrá F, editors. The Encyclopedia of Food and Health. 3rd ed. Oxford: Elsevier Inc.; 2016. pp. 476-481

[12] Morehouse KM. Food irradiation: The treatment of foods with ionizing radiation. Food Testing and Analysis. 1998;**8**(3):9-35

[13] Eustice RF, Bruhn CM. Consumer acceptance and marketing. In: Fan X, Sommers CH, editors. Food Irradiation Research and Technology. 2nd ed. Oxford: Blackwell Publishing; 2013. pp. 173-193

[14] World Health Organization. Food Safety and Nutritional Adequacy of Irradiated Foods. 1st ed. Geneva: WHO; 1994. p. 182

[15] Satin M. Radiation of Food. 1st ed. Zaragoza: Editorial Acribia; 1997. p. 221

[16] Byun MW, Lee JW, Yook HS, Jo C, Kim HY. Application of gamma irradiation for inhibition of food allergy. Radiation Physics and Chemistry. 2002;**63**:369-370

[17] Harder MNC. Effect of gamma radiation on allergenic protein hen eggs [thesis]. Piracicaba: USP; 2009. p. 62

[18] US Food and Drug Administration. Irradiation: A Safe Measure for Safer Iceberg Lettuce and Spinach [Internet]. 2008 [Updated: 2008]. Available from: http://www.fda.gov/downloads/ForConsumers/ConsumerUpdates/UCM143389.pdf [Accessed: February 2017]

[19] Food and Drug Administration. Irradiation in the Production, Processing and Handling of Food [Internet]. 2012 [Updated: 2012]. Available from: https://www.federalregister.gov/documents/2012/11/30/2012-28967/irradiation-in-the-production-processing-and-handling-of-food [Accessed: February 2017]

[20] Bernard H. Food Irradiation [Internet]. 2017 [Updated: 2017]. Available from: http://www.barnardhealth.us/food-irradiation/food-intolerance-and-allergy.html 2017 [Accessed: February 2017]

[21] Jedrychowski L, Wichers HJ. Chemical and Biological Properties for Food Allergens. 1st ed. CRC Press, Boca Raton; 2009. p. 447

[22] Vaz AFM, Costa RMPB, Coelho LCBB, Oliva MLV, Santana LA, Melo AMMA, Correia MTS. Gamma irradiation as an alternative treatment to abolish allergenicity of lectins in food. Food Chemistry. 2011;**124**(4):1289-1295

[23] Lee JW, Seo JH, Kim JH, Lee SY, Kim KS, Byun MW. Changes of the antigenic and allergenic properties of a hen's egg albumin in a cake with gamma-irradiated egg white. Radiation Physics and Chemistry. 2005;**72**:645-650

[24] Lee JW, Lee KY, Yook HS, Lee SY, Kim HY, Jo C, Byun MW. Allergenicity of hen's egg ovomucoid gamma irradiated and heated under different pH conditions. Journal of Food Protection. 2002;**65**:1196-1199

[25] Kim MJ, Lee JW, Yook HS, Lee SY, Kim MC, Byun MW. Changes in the antigenic and immunoglobulin E–binding properties of hen's egg albumin with the combination of heat and gamma irradiation treatment. Journal of Food Protection. 2002;**65**(7):1192-1195

[26] Lee JW, Kim JH, Yook HS, Kang KO, Lee SY, Hwang HJ, Byun MW. Effects of gamma radiation on the allergenic and antigenic properties of milk proteins. Journal of Food Protection. 2001;**64**:272-276

[27] Byun MW, Kim JH, Lee JW, Park JW, Hong CS, Kang IJ. Effects of gamma radiation on the conformational and antigenic properties of a heat-stable major allergen in brown shrimp. Journal of Food Protection. 2000;**63**:940-944

[28] Sofyan R, Soedigdo S. The effect of gamma irradiation on fish transaminase and rhodanese. Journal of the Indonesian Atomic Energy Agency. 1983;**16**(1):75-82

[29] Leszczynska J, Lacka A, Szemraj J, Lukamowicz J, Zegota H. The influence of gamma irradiation on the immunoreactivity of gliadin and wheat flour. European Food Research and Technology. 2003;**217**:143-147